The Complete
Natural Medicine Guide
to
Women's Health

Dr. Sat Dharam Kaur, ND
Dr. Mary Danylak-Arhanic, MD   Dr. Carolyn Dean, ND, MD

Robert
ROSE

Acknowledgments

I'd like to dedicate this book to my mom, Sylvia, who passed away in 1988, and my brother, Jack, who passed away in 1995. They both took the time to listen, care, and exemplify how to live a good life. They also emphasized the importance of giving of oneself to others. Thanks also to my father, Sam, and brother, Robert, who helped me develop a strong work ethic and passion toward my career and personal interests while demonstrating to me in their own ways how to strive for and attain excellence in all that I undertake.

I owe much gratitude to my first running mentors, Dr. Brian Smith, Terry Hamlin, and Ken Kurts for imparting to me, both as a runner and as a coach, many of the training methods and philosophies that I use today. Thanks also Randy Brown, my personal friend and fellow coach, for helping me further refine my coaching skills. I have appreciated his counsel and support over the years, and also with this project.

Thanks to all the runners I've had the pleasure to train with and coach over the past twenty years, including those with the Leukemia and Lymphoma Society's "Team in Training" program, members of the cross country teams at the College of Charleston and North Charleston High School, and visitors/clients of my Web site, State of the Art Marathon Training (*www.marathontraining.com*). You've all taught me more about running and coaching than you can imagine!

While they are no longer with us, Dr. George Sheehan and Dr. Charlie Post each inspired me greatly while teaching me so much about the relationship and delicate balance between running and life.

Thanks to Carlo and Dominique DeVito, Dr. Stephen Pribut, and Bethany Brown for their editorial assistance, journalistic contributions, and support with this book. You guys were great!

And finally, to Susan Ziman, for your love and encouragement. You're the woman I've waited nearly a half-century to accompany me on the long run of life.

Enjoy *The Everything® Running Book* and I'll see you on the roads!

—Art Liberman

Introduction

Why Run?

Running is one of the types of exercise available to all people. And it also has one of the lowest equipment needs of any sport. You don't need a ball, or a field, or an umpire. You don't need a gym or a pool or a track. You might already own everything you need—running shoes, a T-shirt, and a pair of shorts. That's about it.

Sure, there are those runners who go beyond that. Like any other competitive sport, runners have found other gizmos and gadgets like pedometers, fancy warm-up suits, elaborate heart rate monitors with all the bells and whistles, but they aren't essential items for the beginner or novice runner.

The other good thing is that you can run alone or with other people. You can run with friends at the same pace, or you can run competitively with them. You can run with one person, or you can run with a large group. Running is good for the whole family. All ages are encouraged to participate and compete.

And there are runners everywhere. Going on a trip? There are runners all over the United States, Europe, Australia, and South America. You name a place, and surely there's a running club there. Don't know where to go for your next vacation? How about a 5K race in Charleston, South Carolina? How about a five-miler in Chicago? How about a marathon in New York, Boston, Los Angeles, or Hawaii? There are thousands upon thousands of road races from the 5K to the marathon held each year in vacation spots all over the United States and the world.

And that leads to the most important point. Runners are everywhere. And everyone who runs is a runner. What do they call the guy who finishes last in a 5K or a marathon? A runner. How fast you are is not the yardstick by which other runners judge you. In running, it's not you versus the other person. The supreme fascination of running is that it is *you against you!*

Beginning a running program can hold many other benefits, not the least of which is your health. For every hour you run ten-minute miles, you burn 4.2 calories per body pound. Jumping rope is 3.8 calories per body pound, and swimming is 3.5 calories per body pound. Half an hour spent running is like riding a bike for an hour, chopping wood for an hour, playing tennis doubles, or weight training for an hour. Compared to other fitness activities, the time savings running provides is an incredible advantage in this fast-paced life we lead.

Take it from Ed Daley of Freehold, New Jersey: "I began running in 1979. It enabled me to keep my weight down and it improved my quality of life. I enjoyed life more, I wasn't tired, wasn't heavy. I was able to do more things with ease and comfort. Running improved my fitness and my outlook. I felt better about everything."

In this book you'll learn how to stay on track and stay motivated to get to the point where you won't want to miss your runs, either. There's also lots of running-related health and nutritional information. This is very important. Many folks shy away from learning about fitness and the body because they think it is complicated; but we've simplified it for you. Your running will benefit because of it.

Find out for yourself about the new and healthier lifestyle that awaits you. It costs pennies a day and will make a huge impact on your life. The latter is the best reason to run. Enjoy, and good luck!

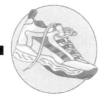

CHAPTER 1

Try It, You'll Like It!

As technological advances such as dishwashers, automobiles, and riding mowers have changed our lifestyles, we have lost something valuable: regular physical work. Because we have mechanized even simple activities that use our arms, legs, back, heart, and lungs, our bodies have become more flaccid, fat, and weak. We are meant to be active, and our health depends upon it. Running is one way to help your body thrive.

Striving for Physical Fitness

Fitness is not a "destination" that you visit occasionally in your life. Rather, fitness is the actual "journey," an ongoing state of health. Participating in a fitness program consistently and regularly may ensure your best chances for improved quality and length of life.

So how do you become fit? As with any project, when you use the right tools, the job is much more productive, efficient, and even fun. The tools for fitness include exercise and nutrition. For us, running will be the exercise of choice. But to get started, we need to begin where all activity originates—in the mind.

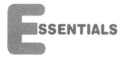
SSENTIALS

Take a minute to write down five reasons why you want to get fit by incorporating running into your life. You may be surprised by your reasons, and they may change over time. Review your answers in one month, then two, to see how far you've gotten.

Getting in the Right Mindset

It may sound funny, but in fact, fitness really does begin in the mind. In order for your body to get moving, your brain needs to have the right mindset. Some of the most common reasons people give for why they don't or shouldn't run are described below. How many do you recognize as ones you've used yourself?

You Don't Have Enough Time

You might think, "I don't have time to run" or "Running is not the most important thing I need to do today." However, you have a choice about how you spend your time. Ask yourself what is the most important thing you need to do today? What is it that you are making time for? Is your health important to you? Keep in mind that out of just about all exercise options, running requires the least amount of time.

You're Worried About How You'll Look

You may also be concerned with how you'll look while running and are worried that you'll look silly. You probably think everyone else who runs looks silly, too, so at least you'll have lots of company! When you're fit and feeling good, though, you won't look or feel silly. Similarly, you may dislike the idea of sweating a lot when you run. Just remember that sweating is a natural bodily function. Be glad your cooling system is working.

You Don't Want to Get Hurt

If you're afraid you'll hurt yourself running, read on. You'll learn exactly what to do from us. Running shouldn't be uncomfortable or hurt when done properly. Through this book, you'll learn what to do safely and systematically and will learn how to achieve a level of running and fitness that is a far safer lifestyle than the one you are currently leading. Finally, don't be concerned that you're too old to run. That was your old life. Start your new life today. No one is too old to run.

You Don't Want to Spend the Money

You may believe that running is expensive and must have some hidden fees or costs. However, running is probably the most inexpensive form of exercise there is. And besides, being unhealthy is more expensive in the long run.

No More Excuses: Time for the New You

There will always be excuses for not doing what you really want to do. You probably recognized many excuses from the above list as reasons you've given in the past not to run. Now is the time to stop making excuses. To get yourself ready to be a runner, you need a new way of thinking about running.

Adjust Your Attitude

First, let go of past ideas about fitness and running. Acknowledge and release old and negative attitudes. They can be unhealthy roadblocks, and they are not useful to you anymore. You have a choice regarding what you think about, so let those negative thoughts go and start anew.

Maybe you think you will never enjoy running. If that's the case, then make peace with it by finding the good in it. Think about some of the benefits it could provide: new friends, improved energy, a better mood, and a healthier lifestyle. As with most runners who persevere from the beginning, you will probably come to love it if you just give it a chance.

The best way to approach running is with an adventurous spirit. When was the last time you tried something new and healthy? Challenge yourself; be a risk taker. And if nothing else works to motivate you, think of the phrase that Nike made famous: "Just do it!"

Make Time to Run

Think of running as a daily, non-negotiable activity. Do you think about whether or not you are going to brush your teeth each day? Your dental hygiene is probably a non-negotiable part of your routine that you wouldn't think of not doing. That is how you should begin thinking about running. It is something to fit into your day.

Consider your running time as a health appointment with yourself. If you had a serious life-challenging illness and through regular treatments you could reclaim your health, wouldn't you plan your time with respect to scheduling and going to those appointments? Well, running is a lifesaving appointment! It helps prevent a variety of sedentary-based conditions, such as cardiovascular disease.

Build a Relationship with Running

Becoming a runner will take more than a short-term commitment. Do most people commit to marriage after the first several dates? No. So like dating, when you begin a running program, don't do it with the end in mind. Add running to your life as you would a long-term relationship: day-by-day. Start out dating, go slowly, and take some time to get to know yourself as a runner. Build a solid relationship with running. You don't start running by doing a marathon. Set as a goal short workouts and be proud of what you accomplish. Learn by taking the small steps, and your relationship with running or walking will be a lifelong love affair.

Focus on the Health Benefits of Running

Turn your view of health inside out. How much time do you spend on exterior appearances such as clothes, hair, nails, and skin? Many people spend more time attending to their exterior appearance than their interior health. The truth is, without your interior health your exterior appearance is meaningless. Next time you look in the mirror, look deeper into your body. Imagine the interior of your body and know that running will improve it. What looks better—a new piece of clothing or how all of your clothes fit after you've lost 5 to 15 percent body fat?

Think of your running time as an investment in your health that will yield invaluable returns. In only one half hour a day (that's less than 2 percent of your whole day!), you can reap tremendous returns. You, not other market considerations, control this investment. Regular running is vital to achieving optimal health while also helping protect you from many preventable diseases. It can be less expensive than what you pay for most life insurance policies, and the benefits are realized while you are alive!

ESSENTIALS

"Being an emergency physician, I encounter my share of stressful days (and nights). I have consistently found, however, that I feel better, perform better, and am actually a more empathetic doctor when I work after running. I am convinced of a neurohumoral response that takes place in my body and which energizes me, yet at the same time settles me and helps me focus, even under harried circumstances."

—Ben Bobrow, Las Vegas, NV

Talk to Other Runners

If you were to ask runners how they feel since including regular exercise in their lives, what would you expect to hear them say? How about the following:

- Running made me feel lethargic, grouchy, and stressed.
- Running made me feel worse about myself.
- Running made me feel and look terrible in my clothes.
- Running made me fatter.
- Running made my sleep patterns poor.
- Running made me start smoking and drinking.
- Running made my blood pressure go up.

Of course not! You probably know that people who run regularly claim just the opposite. They boast renewed energy, a better outlook on life, a tendency to eat healthier foods, better quality of sleep, and more. What is it about running that produces all of these effects? It's the fact that running is a form of aerobic exercise.

Aerobic exercise does for the body what no other activity can because of one major process: the utilization of oxygen. Sure, you take in oxygen all the time just by breathing. But when you run, you take in greater amounts of oxygen and it is delivered more deeply into the body because the heart, lungs, and muscles are working harder. Circulation increases, and with it, oxygen delivery. This is beneficial for your body and makes you feel good.

The body loves regular bouts of oxygen-rich running and, like a welcomed houseguest, makes accommodations for it. The body actually craves a higher aerobic level. These accommodations are the training benefits; they show up in the body not only during exercise but also while at rest. No wonder exercise makes us feel better!

ESSENTIALS

If your friends are runners already, ask them what they like and dislike about running. If they're not runners, ask them if they'd like to be. Recruit one of your non-running friends to start this program with you and share your experiences as you train. You'll double your pleasure and be able to share your joys as well as your challenges.

Benefits of Running

It is highly motivating to know that you are improving yourself on the inside and the outside. Following are some of the more common and well-documented benefits of running. Let's take a look at what's awaiting you!

Physical Benefits of Running

Running helps to improve respiration, making you an "easy breather." When you run, your body needs more oxygen to "fund" the activity. Your lungs work harder than when they are at rest to supply the extra demand for oxygen to the body. With repetition and time, your lungs adapt to the extra workload and become more efficient at providing the extra oxygen needed for the activity. The overall effect of this extra work is that you will experience more efficient and easier breathing at rest as well as when you are active.

Running also improves cardiac output. Just as an assembly line measures success in terms of productivity, or output, cardiac output refers to the productivity of the heart. It is the measure of the heart rate and volume of blood that is pumped out with each heartbeat. When you run, your heart beats at a much faster rate than when you are at rest so that your muscles will receive more blood. The more you run, the stronger and more efficient your heart becomes. The training effect of running upon cardiac output is that the heart rate at rest beats slowly yet is able to pump out large amounts of blood with each beat. You get more output for less effort, improving your heart's efficiency.

As with cardiac output, running also positively affects the vascular system. Blood and oxygen move through our body's "highway system," the vascular system. Through running, veins and arteries become cleaner due to a reduction of fatty deposits. Exercise also increases the number and size of blood vessels, which is the equivalent of having more paved streets in your neighborhood. Travel becomes less congested and laborious, and your circulation and blood pressure are improved.

Additional benefits of running occur with improved muscular strength and endurance. When you run, you use one of the body's major tools:

your muscles. You need muscular strength and endurance in order to perform activity or work. Muscular endurance is your ability to maintain that activity or work over time. One of the effects of running is that it keeps your muscles functional and strong.

Running also contributes to increased bone density. Muscles are attached to bone, so when you move your muscles during running, it is as if the muscles are massaging and tugging on the bones. The training effect upon your bones is growth. Think of muscular movement like a bone massage that stimulates bone growth. Bone growth helps to keep bones dense, firm, and healthy.

In addition to stimulating bone growth, running can also improve the flexibility of your joints. A joint is the place where bones meet. When you have movement of your joints, it feels good; when you cannot move your joints, it feels bad. The training effect of running on your joints is that it helps maintain and improve the mobility or range of motion within a joint.

A benefit of running you may not have thought of is the improvement of bowel function. Running helps to stimulate the wavelike movement in the bowels called *peristalsis*. How does it do this? It can be related to several factors, including pressure changes inside the body as a result of increased breathing, the neighboring muscular movement, or increased gravitational pull of some activities. In addition to having enough fiber and fluid in your dietary intake, movement will help your ability to eliminate. Regular and easy elimination helps prevent hemorrhoids and constipation.

Another physical benefit of running is enhanced sensory skills. As babies and youngsters, we learn how to use our sensory skills. We learn about balance and movement in space through activity. In order to keep these sensory skills sharp, we have to use them. A training effect of running is the maintenance and improvement of sensory skills, like balance and movement through space or from place to place.

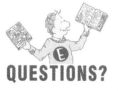

QUESTIONS?

What is meant by the "training effect"?

The training effect is your body's response to a workout. When your body is stressed by exercise, it makes physical adaptations afterward so that it won't be as stressed during future workouts. These are the training effects, the positive changes we associate with exercise!

Psychological Benefits of Running

A well-known training effect of running is the production of endorphins. Endorphins are natural morphine-like hormones that produce a sense of well-being and reduce stress levels. They make you feel good and improve your mood. You may have heard of the "runner's high" associated with long-distance runners, but these runners don't have the exclusive rights to endorphin production. You too can produce your own endorphins, without being a distance runner. Regular exercise will trigger the endorphins' release.

Another improved psychological effect is that running seems to enhance the creative and problem-solving processes for many people. Many people use their daily run as a time to reflect and think through things, plan their days and weeks, or even clear their minds from the pressures of a hectic workday.

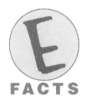

FACTS

"I began running in June of 2000 at a time in my life when I was very depressed and overweight. I knew I had to do something to make my life better. I began running and it changed my life. Since I began running, I have lost fifty-five pounds and my self-esteem and self-confidence levels are very high."

—Danielle Utillo, Staten Island, NY

Social Benefits of Running

We are social animals who enjoy and need human interaction. Running helps you to build self-confidence, which spills into other areas of your life. Don't be surprised if you feel a bit more outgoing and social after beginning your running program; it is another training effect of exercise.

The opportunities for social experiences can be either direct or indirect. You may choose the direct experience of running with others. Or if you prefer running to be time for yourself, you can still indirectly use running as a conversation piece in other professional or social situations.

FACTS

"Camaraderie is one of the main benefits of joining a running club. It gives you the opportunity to socialize and meet other runners. You exchange information, pick up running tips, maybe even find a training partner. You also find out news and information about upcoming events [and] get discounts on club-sponsored races."

—Linda Hyer, Marlboro, NJ,
Freehold Area Running Club President

Your loved ones will also be proud of you for your commitment to running. Suppose someone special says to you, "I started a running program a month ago." How do you respond? Do you reply, "Oh no, how could you do such a thing?" or "Oh, I'm so sorry"? Of course not! You would probably congratulate him or her and offer support. Others will have the same reaction toward you, helping to reinforce your motivation.

You Will Feel Better, Absolutely!

If you somehow were able to achieve those benefits through non-running means—that is, through medical and therapeutic services—you would have had to spend numerous hours and large sums of money, take various types of medications, and deal with the negative side effects. In addition, you would not have much fun in the process, and there are no guarantees that the medical and therapeutic means would work. Running can make you feel better with less expense, less stress, and more fun. Now that you have the right mindset about running, it's time to learn how to be successful in this new undertaking.

ALERT

Everyone begins a fitness program with gusto. But if you do too much too soon, instead of feeling great you'll get hurt. Then you'll feel worse than you might now! Are you physically able to start a running program right now? If you're not sure, check with your doctor.

CHAPTER 2

Setting Yourself Up for Success

Before you trot off to create the new you, there are some basic things you need to know to protect yourself over time. After all, this is not going to be just another hobby started and given up on. It's going to become your way of life.

Choosing a Running Program

In order to come up with a program that will work best for you, you need to be specific about what your needs and goals are. Is your primary goal to lose a certain amount of weight? Be realistic about how long it could take. Do you need to fit running into a very busy schedule? If so, you may only have time for a half hour a day. That's fine! This book will help you optimize the time you do have.

Above all, stick with one program. Don't haphazardly adopt several training plans and jump from one to the other. If possible, find a coach and follow his or her training plan. A qualified coach will consult with you on a regular basis so that, if necessary, your program can be modified should you experience fatigue, soreness, and/or injury.

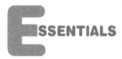

ESSENTIALS

How many times have you intended to change something in your life but it didn't happen? Lots of times, if you're like most people. Well, that's not going to happen this time. You're going to start small, have multiple successes, and stay motivated by the differences in how you look and feel. You can do this by setting realistic, feel-good goals.

The Principles of Successful Running

Not knowing how to start is often the most significant roadblock keeping people from beginning a running program. However, with the right map in hand, you can get started, know where you are going, and enjoy the ride. The following steps will set you up for success. They are the road to fitness and health.

Schedule Running into Your Life

Pull out your daily planner/calendar and look at the week ahead of you. Schedule your exercise session to fit into your busy schedule. Find the desirable time of day or evening to exercise and make it a regular habit.

Arrange for family cooperation if necessary. Perhaps your spouse can trade early morning responsibilities with you; perhaps your children can learn how to make their own breakfast so you can run before taking them to school. When you use your daily planner with an opportunistic eye, you can reserve a small part of your busy days for your exercise time.

Think about ways to include family members if they can't be left alone. Buy a baby jogger or stroller and take your youngster with you. Or allow an older child to ride a bike while you run. A child's designated time for homework can be your designated time for body work.

A frequently asked question is: When is the best time of day to do my bodywork—morning, afternoon, or evening? The best answer is: The time when you will do it. Some people have a regular schedule that makes it easy for them to plan their exercise at a designated time and day. For others, no two days are alike, and they have to create windows of opportunity for exercise time.

We manage to make time every day for the appointments we can't miss. We get to work on time, pick the kids up from school, go to dentist appointments, and set aside time to read the newspaper or talk on the telephone. We find time for these activities because they are important to us. When you have something important in your life, you are more apt to cherish it and treat it with respect.

Schedule your exercise time as you would these other important appointments; keep your appointment, be punctual, and give yourself a start and finish time. A nice side effect to being regular about your exercise time is that those around you (your spouse, partner, boss, children, coworkers, or employees) will learn that exercise time is your private time to be respected and not to be infringed upon unless absolutely necessary.

FACTS

Although exercising is beneficial at any time of the day, many people prefer running in the morning. By doing this, they have the rest of the day to enjoy the energizing effects of their run.

Make Your Runs Fun and Convenient

Invite a friend, neighbor, or coworker to join you as a regular or an occasional workout partner. Make sure you choose someone whose company you enjoy so that you will look forward to sharing that time. Additionally, find someone who is also a beginner so that both of you will be running at the same approximate pace.

Canine companions are also usually happy to be included on jogs. Make sure that if your dog isn't used to running long distances, take extra care in conditioning your pet. You have to remember that his/her paws and cardiovascular system also need time to adapt and adjust. And of course your dog should be one for whom this kind of exercise is possible; you won't get far with a Chihuahua or a Pug, for example.

ALERT

Remember to carry along some water for your canine runner—dogs can overheat quickly. Check out the dog packs that your four-legged friend can carry on his/her back; just remember to keep it light. Also, be considerate of how much running your particular dog can handle.

Wear the Right Clothing

You can also make your runs more enjoyable by investing in elements of exercise that can make you feel good about yourself. For example, whether or not you wear functional and comfortable clothing can make a world of difference as to whether you enjoy or dread working out. Wear workout garb that gives you confidence. If you have been saving your worn-out T-shirts, shorts, and sweats for exercise, think again. Those old clothes may not do much for your motivation, especially if you're a beginner who feels a bit self-conscious about running anyway.

There are many products out in the marketplace that will be especially useful, such as Coolmax and other synthetic blend fabrics that we'll discuss later in the book. These are designed to not only look good, but also to help keep you cool, reduce/eliminate chafing, wick away moisture, and in short, make you feel comfortable.

Start Incrementally and Increase Gradually

When becoming physically active, more is not always better. Before you learned to walk, you had to crawl, and the same is true for your fitness. If you want to be successful with your program and feel good both during and after exercise, you will need to start with small increments of time and effort and then increase gradually.

This is where many people set themselves up to fail. They expect their body to perform at levels that are neither realistic nor recommended. Then afterward they wrongly insist that it's the exercise itself that made them feel that way. The key point here is to be patient and consistent.

It is particularly important to start slowly if you have not exercised recently. When you first begin to move, it is as if your body has been in a coma. If someone was coming out of a coma, would you shake them and say, "Hey, come on, get going, faster, harder, more, more"? Of course not. Similarly, when you begin an exercise program, you should be gentle with your body. If you start slowly, your body will respond favorably.

To set yourself up for success, start with small increments of time at low intensity levels until your body has had time to adjust to the new activity. Understanding and applying some basic principles of fitness will help you achieve your goals. Some people (oftentimes former athletes) may feel embarrassed by running at a slow pace at first. You need to put this concern aside so that you don't set yourself up for injury.

Following basic principles of exercise establishes the foundation for a solid and successful exercise program. These principles are centered around the idea that stressing one's muscles at the appropriate level (the workout) followed by rest leads to the next higher level of fitness. Understanding this idea can help you determine workout specifics such as frequency, intensity, time, and type. By considering these factors, you can optimize your workouts and increase your abilities at a safe and healthy pace.

Fitness expert, author, endurance athlete, and exercise physiologist Sally Edwards reminds us in her book *Smart Heart* that "you can only manage what you can measure and monitor." This is certainly true for exercise and health. If you want to take an active role in your fitness, keep track of what you do, how much you do, and any other interesting pieces of information that relate to your health. You can be as descriptive as you like. You do not have to be obsessive about every detail but should include enough to tell a story about your exercise and health.

FACTS

"After having my second baby, I became frustrated that I had not lost the last ten pounds of baby weight. This is when I found Art Liberman's mileage buildup program. I dedicated myself to, and completed, the nineteen-week program. When I finished the ten-mile run, I felt fabulously proud of myself. My self-confidence and self-image soared."

—Shelley Barineau, Houston, TX

Beyond Motivation: The Basics

The following is a quick overview of the many things you will need to know to get started with your running program so you can train safely and successfully. These topics are explored in depth later in the book, but they're mentioned briefly here to point out some essential things that you must take into consideration when first getting started.

Equipment and Training Log

Buy a new pair of running shoes from someone knowledgeable. The sales staff in specialty running stores are usually runners themselves and have the technical knowledge to put you in the right shoes to meet your biomechanical needs. Don't be afraid to ask questions.

When the mileage totals of your shoes reach a maximum of 400 miles, it's time to buy a new pair. You may think 400 miles sounds like a lot, but as you become a more experienced runner, mileage totals will accrue quickly. Training in shoes that have exceeded their lifespan can lead to a variety of overuse injuries that may take days or weeks to heal properly. When considering clothing (such as socks, shirts, and shorts), choose those manufactured with synthetic blends such as Coolmax that wick away perspiration and reduce the possibility of chafing.

Another item that will improve your running experience is a training log. Use a notebook, calendar, or running log to record at least the following information: miles run, total time run, and shoe model worn. Some runners even record everything from the weather conditions to the route they run to the total shoe mileage.

Keeping a log is important because it provides a history of your running, which can be crucial to finding the possible cause of a running injury. Additionally, reviewing a running log helps determine the training methods that were the most effective regarding one's best performances. Finally, keeping a log is highly motivating, as few runners like to leave too many blank spaces. However, do not become compulsive about your running just to "fill in the blanks" or to reach a specific weekly mileage total, no matter what.

There are a variety of Web sites that provide training logs and show you how to record everything pertaining to your training program, from actual miles run to cumulative shoe mileage. Best of all, most of these Web sites are free! (See Appendix C, "Running Online.")

E **SSENTIALS** A training log may not seem like an essential item in your quest for fitness, but it is! It's a place to set goals, track achievements, and note ups or downs. You'll be thrilled to look back at all that you did, and you'll be more motivated to stick to your plan.

Build a Base

Without question, the most important area one should focus on when beginning a running program is that of safely building a mileage base, or the distance you run per week. It's important to start out with small increments and build on them, no matter how silly or short they might seem. Never try to take on too much too soon. Doing so can greatly increase your chances of incurring an overuse injury and may ruin your appetite for running.

In a chapter all about motivation and success, it's hard not to feel like you can strap on your running shoes and do five miles easily. While it's excellent to want to seize the day, remember, slow and steady wins the race. You'll be doing that easy five miles soon enough if you train smart.

In building your mileage base, remember the 10 percent rule: Do not increase either your weekly mileage and/or long run mileage by more than 10 percent a week. Doing so greatly increases the chances of incurring an injury, thereby delaying or stopping your training altogether. This is one of the biggest mistakes runners make. Don't do it!

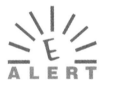

You shouldn't even think of training for a marathon (26.2 miles) until certain conditions have been met. For instance, you should have been running consistently four to five days per week, twenty-five miles per week, for at least a year (without any major injuries).

Nutrition

Nutrition is an essential part of any exercise program and will be covered in greater detail in Chapter 15. One thing to keep in mind at this point, though, is that nutrition is not just about food; it's about fluids, too. Runners must be well-hydrated to run effectively. For runs of up to sixty minutes or less, water is the drink of choice.

It is also important to emphasize healthy foods in your diet and limit fried and high-fat foods. There is much debate now regarding the proper mix of carbohydrates, proteins, and fats. As a runner, you should focus on carbohydrate sources in your diet, aiming for carbohydrates to make up approximately 65 percent of your total daily calories. Split the remaining 35 percent of calories between proteins and fats.

Cross-Training and Weight Training

Without a doubt, runners should include supplemental activities such as weight training and cross-training as part of their total fitness program. In particular, incorporating weight training, stretching, and carefully selected cross-training activities to your fitness regimen both reduce the risk of injury and facilitate total body conditioning. You can read more about weight training and cross-training in Chapter 8.

Common Mistakes

Again, simple, unintentional mistakes are some of the easiest and most common ways for runners to derail their programs. These particular runners can be categorized into two major groups. The first type adopts the philosophy that "more is better" and builds their mileage too rapidly, thus suffering breakdown and/or injury.

The second group of individuals is very inconsistent in their training and may miss several workouts in a row. Then, recognizing that they are behind in their training, they'll add on additional miles in an effort to catch up. Neither approach will help you to become a successful runner. With this book, you can avoid both of these approaches.

Avoiding Injury

One of the greatest challenges of running is to remain injury free. Although some runners may wear their injuries like a badge of honor, more injuries come from not properly training than getting hurt on the course. Just as there are different types of runners, there are many types of injuries and treatments.

If you suspect you may have an injury, begin a preventative rehabilitation program to keep the damage to a minimum. Depending on the type of injury, this might mean using ice, over-the-counter anti-inflammatory medication (such as Aleve and Advil), and above all, taking a rest day or two to allow the injury to heal. Chapter 13 discusses specific ways to greatly reduce your chances of incurring an injury.

FACTS

Should you experience a minor injury while running, apply RICE. No, not the grain, the principle:

R = Rest
I = Ice
C = Compress
E = Elevation

If there's swelling or pain, take an anti-inflammatory, such as aspirin or ibuprofen. If your injury doesn't respond to self-treatment in a couple of days, see a doctor.

Stretch Regularly

Beginning runners often underestimate the value of stretching. Stretching is one of the most effective means of avoiding injury and increasing performance and stamina. However, don't stretch a cold muscle before you exercise. It's much safer to stretch after your workout. If a person really wants to stretch beforehand, he or she should do some brisk walking or a slow ten-minute jog, and then stretch. The necessity and benefits of stretching regularly as part of your workout routine, let alone any more-ambitious training program, cannot be overemphasized.

Utilize Recovery Techniques

There are several therapeutic measures you can take to recover from stressful workouts or from the cumulative effects of hard training over a long period of time. Massage therapy, for example, feels great after a long run, hard race, and/or weeks of heavy training. Another therapeutic technique is pouring cold water on fatigued legs after a race or long workout. You can also try soaking your legs in a whirlpool of warm water (approximately 105 degrees Fahrenheit) a couple of hours after working out. Something as simple as taking a walk or going for an easy bike ride a couple hours after a hard workout can also do wonders for tired legs.

CHAPTER 3
The Well-Equipped Runner

Running is one of the least equipment-intensive sports you can participate in. In fact, all you really need to run are shorts, a shirt, and shoes. But if you're going to do it right, you need to know that not just any shorts, shirts, or shoes will do. Appropriate gear should be comfortable and assist you in staying injury-free.

Running Shoes

First, you need to outfit your feet with running shoes. These should not be just any running shoes; they should be running shoes that meet your particular biomechanical needs. Take advantage of the fact that running shoes are designed to minimize injury and maximize form and function.

There are three factors to consider in determining the best type of shoe for a particular runner. The first involves what foot type the runner has (high arch, flat foot, or normal arch). It's also important to analyze the runner's footstrike (heel striker, forefoot striker, or midfoot striker) and stride pattern (pronater, supinater, or neutral). Footstrike and stride pattern will be discussed in detail in Chapter 4.

Buying Running Shoes

To be sure all of these considerations are met when buying your shoes, you should purchase your shoes at a specialty running store rather than at a wholesale sporting goods store. Specialty running stores are places that cater to the needs of runners. Often owned by runners themselves, these stores employ knowledgeable individuals who understand shoe construction and are familiar with the latest models and brands on the market. In short, the staff of specialty running stores are experts in matching your particular foot type and stride pattern to the specific shoe that will best meet your biomechanical needs.

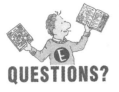

QUESTIONS?

Is there a "best" time of the day to try on running shoes?
When shoe shopping, you can get the best and most comfortable fit for your feet by going later in the day when your feet have swelled to their maximum size.

It is also important to remember that there may be several types/models of running shoes among various brand names (Nike, Saucony, New Balance, Brooks, etc.) that will meet your biomechanical needs. In other words, don't assume that only one brand will work for you.

When trying on running shoes, try them on with the style sock or one of similar thickness to the socks you will wear when running. When standing in the shoes, you should have a distance equal to the width of your thumb between your longest toe and the end of the shoe. Improperly fitting shoes without enough room between your longest toe and the front of the toebox can lead to black toenails or toenails that fall off. Additionally, your heels should not slip out of the back of the shoes when you walk or run in them.

Since you will be doing more than standing in your running shoes, you will want to run around in them before making your purchase. If the store has space, run around inside, getting off the carpet and onto a hard surface. However, don't run outside with them unless you've asked permission first.

If the store won't let you run in them, make sure it has a good return policy. Otherwise, shop at another store. Don't be one of those people, though, who takes advantage of a return policy by bringing back shoes that have been worn for several workouts.

FACTS

Base your decision to purchase new running shoes on the number of miles your old pair has on them, not by observing how much tread remains on the outersole. The midsole of many running shoes breaks down between 350 and 500 miles and offers little or no protection after that period of time.

Types of Running Shoes

Most beginners, as well as people of average to heavy weight, will need shoes that provide support, cushioning, and shock absorption. The lighter training shoes (lighter in weight than most running shoes, that is) are designed for experienced runners for their fast-paced workouts and races. These shoes can also be used by some lighter-weight runners. Because they weigh less than most running shoes, they can help shave a few seconds off one's pace. However, due to their lighter weight, they don't offer quite the same degree of protection as a traditional training shoe.

Racing flats are similar to light-weight trainers but are even lighter in weight and thus offer less protection. They should be used only by the advanced competitor for fast-paced, short-distance training sessions, along with shorter races.

When selecting a shoe, remember also that shoe companies work hard to get your attention. Their designs and colors are meant to attract you so that you will buy their shoes. However, resist buying a particular style of running shoe because you want to make a fashion statement. You will do yourself a big favor if you think about function over fashion.

The Parts of a Running Shoe

Oftentimes when shopping for footwear, a salesperson will use high-tech words to describe the particular features and parts of the running shoe. With a little basic knowledge of running shoes, you can become a more informed buyer and satisfied user. This shoe anatomy session can help you buy the shoe that's right for you.

The toebox refers to the toe section of the shoe. It should be roomy enough to comfortably fit your toes. There should be approximately a half an inch between your longest toe and the end of the shoe, and a half an inch between the top of your longest toe and the top of the toebox.

Next, take a look at shoe laces. You should use laces that are not too long or too slippery. If they are too long, cut them down and/or use lace locks.

ALERT

Occasionally, runners complain about their feet feeling tingly or numb, particularly during longer training runs. This can sometimes be attributed to shoe laces being tied too tightly, which reduces the circulation of blood to one's feet. A simple solution for this annoying problem is to tie your laces just tightly enough so that your shoes stay snugly on your feet.

Held together by the laces is the upper, or the material that encloses the foot. Breathable fabrics such as mesh keep feet from overheating in the summer. When choosing a shoe, be sure the upper fits properly; it helps the shoe stabilize the foot.

Beneath the laces you will find the tongue of the shoe. The tongue should be thick enough to protect the top of the foot from pressure of the laces, but not so long that it rubs against your foot just above the ankle.

Several parts of the shoe are designed around its heel. At the back of the shoe is the heel notch, the slight depression cut into the shoe's heel collar to reduce Achilles-tendon irritation and provide a more secure heel fit. The heel counter is the rounded place where your heel fits snugly yet comfortably. Too loose a fit can cause blisters on your heels. If you need extra stability (for instance, your feet wobble a lot), look for a stiff heel counter or an external heel counter (a ring that wraps around the outside of the heel). On the bottom of the shoe, look for the split heel, a two-part heel structure that separates the outer and inner sides and contributes to a smoother heel-to-toe transition.

Look for heel heights that match your cushioning needs. If you are a big person, chances are you are more of a heel-striker and want more midsole foam under the heel, so you need a greater heel height. Faster runners tend to strike more in the mid-foot and need a lower heel.

Most of the cushioning and shock absorption in shoes is provided by the midsole, the part of the shoe that you can't see (located above the outersole). You will want one of two midsole foams: polyurethane or EVA. Polyurethane is denser, heavier, and more durable than EVA. EVA is a softer, cushier material. Generally, heavier runners do well with polyurethane midsoles. EVA is more common because of its lightness and more cushioned feel.

The material that covers the bottom of the shoe is referred to as the outersole. You will want one of three kinds of outersole: carbon rubber, blown rubber, or a combination of the two. Carbon rubber is more durable but heavier and stiffer than blown rubber. Some shoes have carbon rubber in the high-wear areas of the rearfoot and the cushier blown rubber in the forefoot for a softer feel.

Running shoes also contain stabilizing technology, or devices that reduce overpronation. These are usually in the shoe's midsole on the arch side of the shoe. Some shoes have firmer densities of midsole foam to combat overp ronation. Pronation and overpronation will be discussed in greater detail in Chapter 4.

Wearing and Caring for Your Running Shoes

One important aspect of wearing running shoes to consider is how you lace them. Lacing your shoes may sound like a silly thing to discuss, but how you do it can make a tremendous difference in how your feet feel in the shoes. Does your heel slip in your shoes? Does the top of your foot get irritated or fall asleep? If so, the following lacing remedies should help you.

For heel slippage, if your heel moves side to side or up and down, try using the shoe's "lace lock." It will bring the heel of the shoe closer to your heel, alleviating the slipping. If the top of your foot falls asleep or gets irritated, you may have a high instep. A high instep causes your foot to take up an excessive amount of space in your shoe. However, if your foot slides around in your shoe and tightening your laces doesn't fix the problem, you may have a narrow foot. In this case, purchase shoes from manufacturers who offer width sizing options.

ESSENTIALS

When you really get serious about running, consider purchasing two pairs of running shoes rather than just one. By alternating their use every other day, you will increase the life expectancy of each pair and save yourself time with less trips to the shoe store.

Take care of your running shoes and they will take care of you. It's very important to make sure you keep you shoes in the best possible condition. Worn-out shoes can lead to unwelcome aches and pains or even injury. Follow some of these rules, and your feet and legs will thank you for it:

- Wear your running shoes only for running—they will last much longer.
- If your shoes become dirty, hand-wash them with commercial shoe care products rather than machine washing and drying them.
- When your running shoes become wet, stick crumpled-up newspaper inside them to accelerate the drying time.

Running Socks

A general rule for choosing socks is that activities that produce a lot of foot friction require a thicker sock. For example, sports like basketball and racquetball generate a lot of friction and warrant thicker socks. Unless you are running trails (which can create high friction), you can be comfortable running in a thin sock but, again, go with what feels good to you.

There are numerous synthetic fabrics being used today that make socks fit, hold up, and wick away moisture (so that you don't have wet feet, which can cause blisters) better than ever before. There is also no need to suffer with socks that bunch and slip down into your shoes. These will only irritate you while running and may produce some nasty blisters.

Some people tend to take socks for granted, but it only takes one blister to bring your feet to your attention. The fit of your socks can make a tremendous difference in your exercise comfort. Your socks should not constrict your skin or make a deep imprint upon it, especially at the ankles or calves. Socks are meant to support, reduce friction, regulate foot temperature, and promote comfort and circulation, not restrict it. Your socks should not bunch up inside your shoes or slide off your feet, and you should be able to move your feet and wiggle your toes comfortably. Whether you're running simply for overall fitness or to complete a marathon, you can help ensure a pain-free running experience by experimenting with a variety of sock styles until you find the type that best works for you.

Athletic Supporters, Jock Straps, and Compression Shorts

Personal preference will dictate the use of these invaluable protective and supportive devices for boys and men. For contact activities (martial arts) and even some non-intentional contact sports (soccer), athletic cups and supporters may be preferred. None of these is really necessary for running. However, support for men is still a big issue. Two garment styles that have taken the place of the more traditional supporters are running shorts with built-in liners and compression shorts. They reduce movement and vibration, which leads to greater comfort.

Sports Bras

Unlike male support mechanisms, which have been around a long time, sports bras were first introduced in the late 1970s. They didn't become widely accepted until the 1980s, though, when the real running boom hit. One of the original sports bras, called the Jog Bra, defines the category for many people, but all sports bras provide support and comfort for female athletes.

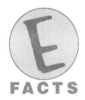

FACTS

In July 1999, American soccer player Brandi Chastain's winning penalty kick gave her team the World Cup Championship. Chastain, in pure ecstasy, spontaneously pulled off her jersey, revealing her sports bra. For that moment, the sports bra was on center stage like never before. Chastain's moment of celebration was captured on the cover of *Newsweek* with the caption, "Girls Rule!"

There are three types of sports bras: compression, encapsulation, and combination. Compression-style bras use the pressure of the fabric to squeeze or press the breasts flat against the chest, limiting movement. This style is favored by small- to medium-breasted women. The encapsulation style limits movement by surrounding and supporting the breasts with reinforced seams or wire (like an underwire bra). This style is preferred by larger-breasted women. The combination style "combines" compression and encapsulation.

There are many options for sports bras, and women are all healthier and happier for them. Comfort should ultimately dictate a woman's choice. The options include underwire, wireless, rear clasp, front clasp, no clasp, front zipper, cross-over-the-head, cross-in-the-back, cross-in-the-front, halter style, nursing compatible, prosthetic compatible, heart rate monitor encapsulable, high impact, and low impact. Fabrics include Lycra,

Coolmax, Supplex, polyester/Lycra, Drylete, cotton, spandex, and mesh. Most of these bras also come in a variety of great colors and styles.

A Running Watch

You will come to depend on your running watch the way you depend on your wristwatch when you think you might be late for work. Your running watch will let you know how you're doing at all times.

The watch you use doesn't have to be expensive (though it can be). Before purchasing a watch for running, decide what functions you think you'll really use. Most include a stopwatch, an alarm, lap settings (also called split timing), a glow light for seeing your time at night, and a regular watch. Make sure the model you choose isn't too complicated or intimidating. The stopwatch will be the part you use most, so make sure it's easy to start, stop, and reset, and is also waterproof.

Other Running Necessities

Depending on the weather and how comfortable you'll be wearing them, you might want to run with one or more of the following: sunglasses, a sweatband, a baseball cap, a wool hat, gloves, and a key/change carrier that can be wrapped around your wrist, ankle, or waist. If you run at night, you'll need reflective gear (or you can sew or glue reflective tape to your gear). Also, don't forget sunscreen when you're out during the day. You'll need it in the winter as much as the summer.

The Runner's Log

How does a training log qualify as equipment? Because without it, you're running in the dark. As we discussed in Chapter 1, there are three main reasons for keeping a log. First, the log provides a history of your running, crucial to finding a possible cause of a running injury. Second, reviewing a running log helps determine the training methods that were the most effective regarding one's best performances. Finally, keeping a log is highly motivating, as few runners like to leave too many empty spaces. (See **TABLE 3-1** for an example log.) Additionally, it's a great idea to keep a shoe mileage chart (see **TABLE 3-2**), which makes it easy to determine when it's time to purchase a new pair of shoes (preferably, when your shoes reach no more than 400 miles).

What to Log

At a minimum, you need to record the distance you actually covered in your workout. This total should also include your warm-up and cool-down mileage because, after all, you did cover that distance on foot. It's really not necessary to measure the road mileage with the odometer of your car, a pedometer, or a cyclo-computer on your bike. You certainly can if you wish to, but that takes away from the spontaneity of your workout.

Running the same routes day after day, week after week, can become boring. I suggest estimating your average pace per mile running by time rather than by mileage. To do this, you can visit a track and run four laps at a relaxed pace (four times around most high school or college tracks equals 1,600 meters, or very close to a mile). You then can run for a specific amount of time and determine the mileage covered. For example, if your easy pace for a mile is nine minutes, run for a little over thirty-six minutes and call the workout a four-miler.

The next item that should be logged is the time duration of your workout. In other words, determine how many total minutes you were moving and running, walking, or a combination of both. If you are using the run/walk method of training, you can be even more specific if you like by recording the actual minutes you were running and the minutes you were walking.

TABLE 3-1.	**RUNNER'S LOG**								
WEEK OF		SUN.	MON.	TUES.	WED.	THURS.	FRI.	SAT.	TOTAL
__/__ TO __/__	TIME								
	MILEAGE								
__/__ TO __/__	TIME								
	MILEAGE								
__/__ TO __/__	TIME								
	MILEAGE								
__/__ TO __/__	TIME								
	MILEAGE								
__/__ TO __/__	TIME								
	MILEAGE								
__/__ TO __/__	TIME								
	MILEAGE								
__/__ TO __/__	TIME								
	MILEAGE								
__/__ TO __/__	TIME								
	MILEAGE								
__/__ TO __/__	TIME								
	MILEAGE								
__/__ TO __/__	TIME								
	MILEAGE								
__/__ TO __/__	TIME								
	MILEAGE								

TABLE 3-2.

SHOE MILEAGE CHART

PAIR #1 _____   ## PAIR #2 _____   ## PAIR # 3 _____

DATE	D.M.	C.M.	DATE	D.M.	C.M.	DATE	D.M.	C.M.
DATE	D.M.	C.M.	DATE	D.M.	C.M.	DATE	D.M.	C.M.
DATE	D.M.	C.M.	DATE	D.M.	C.M.	DATE	D.M.	C.M.
DATE	D.M.	C.M.	DATE	D.M.	C.M.	DATE	D.M.	C.M.
DATE	D.M.	C.M.	DATE	D.M.	C.M.	DATE	D.M.	C.M.
DATE	D.M.	C.M.	DATE	D.M.	C.M.	DATE	D.M.	C.M.
DATE	D.M.	C.M.	DATE	D.M.	C.M.	DATE	D.M.	C.M.
DATE	D.M.	C.M.	DATE	D.M.	C.M.	DATE	D.M.	C.M.
DATE	D.M.	C.M.	DATE	D.M.	C.M.	DATE	D.M.	C.M.
DATE	D.M.	C.M.	DATE	D.M.	C.M.	DATE	D.M.	C.M.
DATE	D.M.	C.M.	DATE	D.M.	C.M.	DATE	D.M.	C.M.
DATE	D.M.	C.M.	DATE	D.M.	C.M.	DATE	D.M.	C.M.
DATE	D.M.	C.M.	DATE	D.M.	C.M.	DATE	D.M.	C.M.
DATE	D.M.	C.M.	DATE	D.M.	C.M.	DATE	D.M.	C.M.
DATE	D.M.	C.M.	DATE	D.M.	C.M.	DATE	D.M.	C.M.
DATE	D.M.	C.M.	DATE	D.M.	C.M.	DATE	D.M.	C.M.
DATE	D.M.	C.M.	DATE	D.M.	C.M.	DATE	D.M.	C.M.
DATE	D.M.	C.M.	DATE	D.M.	C.M.	DATE	D.M.	C.M.
DATE	D.M.	C.M.	DATE	D.M.	C.M.	DATE	D.M.	C.M.
DATE	D.M.	C.M.	DATE	D.M.	C.M.	DATE	D.M.	C.M.
DATE	D.M.	C.M.	DATE	D.M.	C.M.	DATE	D.M.	C.M.
DATE	D.M.	C.M.	DATE	D.M.	C.M.	DATE	D.M.	C.M.

KEY: D.M. = DAILY MILEAGE
      C.M. = CUMULATIVE MILEAGE

For runners who rotate two or more pairs of running shoes for their training from day to day, or even if you own just one pair, it's also important to write down the shoe model you used for your workout and the respective miles run in that particular shoe. This will enable you to track its wear. Many injuries can be traced to training shoes that are worn out.

Other things you can record include, but are not limited to, heart rate (for those runners who use a monitor before and during exercise), weather (temperature, wind, conditions), the specific route you ran, how your legs felt during and after the workout, other cross-training activities done that day, and so on. The key is to have an understanding of what you are willing to record on a day-by-day basis. Some people will want to keep those things simple (recording just mileage, duration, and shoes worn), as they may or may not enjoy or have the time to keep very detailed records.

What to Use as a Training Log

To log the information you choose to record, you can keep things very simple and use a blank calendar or a spiral notebook. *Runner's World* puts out a comprehensive training log that you can use to record your workouts for the entire year. There are also a variety of free Web sites that will enable you to record the specifics of your workout (mileage, shoes, duration, and so on). In short, the choice is yours! Find a system that works easily for you and make sure that you log your workout each and every day.

Using a Calendar

Another way to keep a log is by using a calendar. This can sometimes be better than a separate log because you can also use it to record other events in your life. This gives you an understanding of how other events can be distractions or hindrances to your running. One drawback to calendars is that they are not always easy to write on and don't offer the space to write more extensive notations. Even so, calendars are easy to maintain and give you the opportunity to make running part of your everyday life.

Use It or Lose It

You can have the trendiest gear and the most elaborate log money can buy, but if you don't use any of it, so what? Don't get so focused on how you look that you forget that your equipment has got to be practical. It has to be easy to care for, easy to take on and off, easy to wash, durable, and comfortable. Don't get discouraged if you're not ready to bare all and work out in your sports bra and shorts (women) or in just shorts (men). You will get to that comfort level eventually by thinking positively, continuing to visualize your fitness goals, and, most of all, by putting your equipment to use as you stick to your running program.

CHAPTER 4

The Mechanics of Running

I s there really a right way to run? Conversely, is there really a wrong way to run? The answer to both questions is "yes." However, that does not mean that everyone should run in the same way with the same form. The fact is that form varies from runner to runner. Every person's form emerges naturally over time.

Assessing Running Form

Many of the fastest runners are not necessarily those that are naturally gifted. They don't have to be exceptionally tall or long-limbed. Instead, the best runners are those with economical strides and who run with purpose, power, and determination. Not only can good form can make the difference between running pain-free and running with pain, but good form can also shave minutes off of your running times.

Improving one's speed poses the greatest challenge for a runner. Many runners (both beginners and intermediates) lean forward and run on their toes to try to go faster. This is a sprinting technique. Trying to run a 5K or 10K in this manner will probably result in pain and may even lead to injury. Additionally, running in this way may hinder a runner from achieving his or her fastest possible pace.

Speed can also be affected by bouncing. Bouncing slows the runner down and is extremely inefficient. It creates greater impact on the legs, especially the knees. Bouncers tend not to pick their knees up very high and sometimes swing their legs in an excessive and thus inefficient manner, possibly leading to pain or injury.

There are many other problems regarding form that plague runners. Many of these problems are not readily recognizable. However, once recognized, they are easily corrected. You don't have to have perfect form but even a minor adjustment or modification can make a tremendous difference in your running efficiency and comfort level. Additionally, tweaking your form a bit can reduce your chances of incurring an injury.

The next time you go to a 5K road race or a popular running trail, you should stop and check out the other runners. You can probably tell good form from improper/inefficient form just by watching. How? The runners with good form will appear more graceful; they'll have an economy of movement and a certain style that seems natural and easy, while incorporating good mechanics.

While watching them, take note of what they are doing. Is their forward motion smoother than yours? Are they carrying their arms lower than you? Are they running less on their toes? Are they running with better posture? This is an excellent way to learn through observation and contemplate improving your overall mechanics.

Style and Mechanics

Whether you begin with the right mechanics or not, your first steps running are a natural movement. Running is an action that we have done before. Your running style refers not to wearing the most current fashions, such as the best runner's watch, the most expensive shoes, or the most fashionable new clothing. Style is how you run.

Beginning runners should try running as naturally as possible. They shouldn't force anything. After you've been running for a few months, it's a good idea to get an experienced runner, or preferably a coach, to point out and correct some, if any, of your form flaws/deficiencies. This, in turn, will improve your overall mechanics and running efficiency.

While you want to run naturally, you should keep in mind the proper mechanics. Those mechanics, explained below, if maintained will lead to more efficient form. Don't push yourself to run fast right away. Concentrate first on comfort and form. The way to approach running as a new way of life is to learn the right habits and then perfect them. Even great athletes tweak their form and mechanics continuously throughout their athletic careers.

ESSENTIALS

Things to keep in mind when you run:

- Run relaxed: Tension saps energy and causes fatigue to set in earlier.
- Run naturally: Develop your own running style, while still employing the principles of good running techniques and mechanics.
- Run tall: Good posture while you run creates other good habits like knee lift, natural extension of stride, and better breathing.

The mechanics are the individual functions of the body during running. The main mechanics include breathing; footstrike, also referred to by some as "footprint"; stride; arms and hands, or armstride; and posture, or body angle. Each of these individual areas can affect your efficiency, your comfort, and your results.

While we cannot change completely the way in which we run and we cannot change our bone and muscle structure, we can at least make an effort to become smoother, more efficient runners by attempting to correct the bad habits we may have developed unknowingly. By knowing what the basics of good running technique are, we will possess an understanding of sound biomechanical principles and the techniques we can use to improve our running form.

Breathing

One of the most vital yet underrated things that you can work on to improve your running efficiency is correct breathing technique. Proper breathing is something that needs to be fully understood and practiced. The problem is that many people breathe from their chest rather than from their abdominal region while they run.

Chest breathers have good lungs but may have some trouble breathing while running. One of the secrets to breathing better when you run is to remember to put a little more force into your exhalation. Your body will naturally inhale to make up for this. This will improve your breathing efficiency.

Don't worry if you think you're making too much noise with your breathing while you are running. You may wheeze, snort, cough, or grunt. As long as you're not overexerting yourself, these noises are harmless.

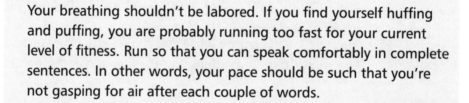

Your breathing shouldn't be labored. If you find yourself huffing and puffing, you are probably running too fast for your current level of fitness. Run so that you can speak comfortably in complete sentences. In other words, your pace should be such that you're not gasping for air after each couple of words.

Establishing Your Breathing Rhythm

Your breathing rhythm is a very important thing. Whether you take three strides for every breath or two strides for every breath, your breathing and your stride are probably in sync naturally. Beginning runners, though, make the mistake of breathing at a 1:1 rate. This means that they are taking one step while breathing in and one step while breathing out. This is essentially panting, and it is inefficient breathing.

The more economical way to breathe depends to a large degree on the pace at which you are running: for your average run, you can breathe 2:2 (taking two steps for every breath in and two steps for every breath out) or 3:3 for longer, slower runs. As you run faster, you may have to breathe more often, which leads to such variations as 2:1 and 1:2 patterns. It's very individualized and it gets you out of the rapid breathing mode and into a rhythm that is more controlled, efficient, and comfortable.

Abdominal Breathing

Whether you're a true beginner or an experienced runner, take the time and effort to learn and employ the abdominal breathing method. Rhythm and stride are closely related to your breathing, so make this a top priority as you progress through your training program. At the very minimum, just remember to keep breathing deep and regularly. In most cases, your breathing will take care of itself; as you run faster, you'll breathe faster. And yes, most runners are mouth breathers or at least nose and mouth breathers. It would be impossible to take in adequate oxygen just breathing through your nose.

Footstrike

Footstrike, or "footprint," is how your foot actually strikes the ground. The footprint is what you leave behind. Each footstrike is like your signature as a runner. Do you run on your toes? Do you run heel-to-toe? Do you run flat footed? The way your foot strikes or comes into contact with the ground is very important. Although you probably cannot change your footstrike significantly, minor adjustments made to correct faulty foot mechanics will enable you to run more efficiently. These corrections include being fitted for the proper shoe to match your foot or possibly adding an orthotic or arch support to your shoe. This, in turn, reduces your chances of incurring an injury.

FACTS

Studies have shown that short- and middle-distance runners first strike the ground with the ball of the foot rather than midfoot or between midfoot and heel. Beginning and intermediate runners should use the heel-ball foot strike (described on pages 42–43), as it allows for better shock absorption, less stress on the calf muscle and Achilles tendon, and better rolling and push-off to the next stride.

Footstrike Types

There are three basic types of footstrikes: normal/neutral, overpronated, and supinated (also called underpronated). In the normal, or neutral, footstrike, the foot rolls slightly inward as it strikes. Your foot flattens out as it makes full contact with the ground, then "rolls" inward to the center of the body. This inward roll of your foot while running, called pronation, is actually a good thing, as it absorbs some of the force that is placed on the foot during the normal exercise of running.

Overpronation occurs when the foot rolls excessively inward upon contact and oftentimes is seen in those who have flat feet. Running shoe models designed and constructed with motion control or stability features help reduce the degree of overpronation. This in turn helps prevent a wide array of overuse injuries that can occur if overpronation is left unchecked.

Supination occurs when the foot doesn't roll inward enough upon hitting the ground and is characteristic of runners with high arches. This minimizes the ability of the foot and in turn, legs, to absorb shock, which can also lead to a host of injuries. To counteract supination, runners with this type of footstrike should wear running shoes that are well-cushioned and flexible.

The Toes' Role in Footstrike

Regardless of what kind of footstrike you have, there are some other things to keep in mind—namely your toes. If it is not totally awkward for you, try to run with your toes pointed forward. Sometimes, especially when we are tired, our feet don't always point forward when we run. In order to get the most power and efficiency from your push-off, work on keeping your feet pointed straight ahead as you run. Doing so results in greater efficiency, which, in turn, enables you to run faster with the same cardiovascular effort. In short, toes and feet that aren't pointed in the right direction result in wasted and inefficient motion.

Of course, this advice is given for those who need to adjust faulty technique in order to improve their form and thus reduce their chances of injury. Some runners are not put together in a way that allows them to have a "perfect" footfall. For those people, a forced effort to run a certain way may actually create a problem worse than just having bad running form.

Another thing to focus on while running is to try to make sure your toes are the last thing off the ground. This will enable you to achieve more power from your stride, resulting in more forward momentum. One's footstrike should be a singular springing motion that is fluid and graceful, resulting in a balanced impact and a powerful push-off.

ESSENTIALS   One way to become more aware of your footstrike is to go for a run paying particular attention to it. Run naturally and, if possible, run past of some windows so you can see your reflection. This will allow you to adjust any flaws you see with your form or posture, which will make you a more efficient runner.

Flat, Heel, and Toe Footstrikes

Many beginners run with a flat footstrike, characterized by landing on a flat foot and having little or no push off. This isn't particularly bad or wrong. If this is the way you run, especially in the beginning, don't change it. Run naturally. To improve your speed and overall efficiency/performance, however, you will need to eventually make some adjustments to your footstrike and push off. These will be discussed later in this chapter.

Other than the flat footstrike, the heel strike is the most common footstrike of beginning runners. With a heel strike, your heel lands first, then you roll along the outer border of your foot until your midfoot makes contact with the ground. Your toes then make contact with the ground as your heel lifts up, and eventually the foot comes off the ground. Again, if this is how you run, you should not change this, especially when you first begin a running program. It is a very normal and natural footstrike.

The heel strike technique is perfectly fine for longer, slower running. However, as with the flat footstrike, to gain speed and efficiency that shorter runs and races require, you may need to move more to the mid-foot strike footprint.

Many beginners "stomp" when they run, hitting too hard with their feet. To keep from becoming this type of runner, try not to make a dent in the earth when you run. Your heel should land gently on the ground. If your feet are slapping the ground and making an audible noise even if you're striking with your heel first, you need to make some serious changes. Land gently on your heel and then roll your foot forward to the mid-foot and then the toes, where you can then push off.

Another type of footstrike is the toe strike. This is a footstrike where only your toes and mid-foot make contact with the ground. This is a sprinting technique and is not appropriate for distance running. Therefore, unless you are a sprinter, don't purposely try running on your toes.

FACTS

In an attempt to improve their speed, many beginning runners compensate by employing either the heel or toe footstrike method. Over time, both methods increase the wear and tear on one's legs, so try to avoid them if at all possible.

Heel-Ball and Ball-Heel-Toe Footstrikes

The preferred method of footstrike for the beginner, intermediate, and heavier runner is the heel-ball strike. In this method, the ball of your foot starts at the deep base of your big toe and goes across your foot to your smallest toe. Although the heel-ball footstrike is where the heel strikes first, it is almost simultaneous with the lowering of the ball of the foot. This footstrike allows for minimum impact over a long period of time, yet has enough push off to generate speed.

A more advanced footstrike technique is the ball-heel-toe strike: For this technique, you land on the outside edge of the ball of your foot, bring your foot down so your heel touches the ground, and then roll back up to push off with your big toe. This technique is for advanced runners because if, as a beginner, you're still in the process of developing the musculoskeletal components in your legs, you will be increasing your risk of injury by employing this footstrike style. The ball-heel-toe footstrike is appropriate to use when you can average under seven minutes per mile in a 5K.

Stride

Stride is how your legs swing into position as you run. Some people have long loping strides, while others have short economical ones. Some lift their knees high, while others barely lift them at all. Stride can make a huge difference in how well you run. Most runners who want to increase their speed turn to adjusting their stride as one of the first places to find the speed they need to make it to the next level.

Start with your natural stride and see where it takes you. Don't be concerned about trying to run fast when you first begin a running program. As beginning runners progress through the first few months of their running program and want to improve their efficiency and speed, there are three adjustments that can be considered: stride frequency, stride length, and knee lift.

ALERT

While it has always been considered a good thing to have a little bounce in your step, in running circles it is a sign that something is wrong. Don't bounce or bound; it means that you are overstriding. If you shorten your stride and eliminate bouncing, you conserve energy that can be better used to propel yourself forward.

Stride Length

Stride length refers to how far you are stepping out when you extend your leg and foot. Increasing your stride length will increase the amount of ground you cover with each step. However, make sure not to overextend your stride, as this too is inefficient.

A good rule of thumb is that you don't want your heel striking the ground too far in front of your knee. Some running experts feel that a short stride is a sign of inflexibility. This is not always so. Proper stretching after a run can help to improve your flexibility, which can lengthen your stride.

Overstriders are easy to spot, as they usually have an excessive kick or rarely bend their knees. They tend to lope or bounce, and their motion is not rhythmic or fluid. Overstriding can actually slow you down due to feet being in contact with the ground longer than with a normal stride length. Make sure that you don't overstride, for this can lead to a host of problems including Achilles tendonitis, iliotibial band pain, and iliopsoas muscle pain.

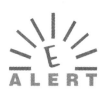

Don't kick your legs up when you run. Some runners kick their heels way up behind them when they run, wasting motion and energy. To get the optimum power from your stride, you should extend your leg behind you when pushing off, and then, bring it forward as soon as possible.

Stride Frequency

Increasing the frequency of your stride is a little more challenging than increasing its length. You're asking your body to move faster than it already is, which isn't an easy thing to do. Basically, you are asking your body to quicken its natural rhythm. One way to improve your stride frequency is by concentrating on your knee motion.

Knee Lift

By focusing on your knee motion, you'll probably improve both your stride frequency and length. Because how far you bring your knees up determines how long your stride will be, you should be careful not to bring your knees up too high. Remember, too long or too short of a stride is inefficient. Therefore, the correct knee lift coupled with the correct frequency of leg turnover will dictate how effectively you can cover ground. In short, the knees do not have to come up very high for long-distance runners. Only sprinters or those charging up a hill have to lift their legs a bit higher than usual.

Arms and Hands

The way you carry your arms helps to provide balance and power while running. Many feel that there is a correlation between moving your arms faster and getting your legs to move faster. Optimally, the arms should support the energy of the body in a forward motion while running.

Your arms provide balance in the following way: as your left leg goes forward, so does your right arm. This balances you as you move forward. Then when the right leg moves forward, so does the left arm. How you carry your arms while moving is called arm carriage.

To have proper arm carriage, your hands should be shaped in a fist, lightly clasped rather than tightly clinched. Don't waste muscle power needlessly. This isn't a stress test, so relax. Leave your fists slightly open and, as you move, allow your arms to swing, carrying them at your side somewhere between your waist and your chest. Make sure they are not too high or too low. One arm swings forward while the other one goes backward in conjunction with the opposite foot and leg motion.

Different types of runners have different types of arm carriage. Sprinters move their arms in a straight forward-backward motion. Most longer distance runners use a slight arc as they swing their arms, but the faster, more efficient ones don't waste motion by moving too much from side to side. In other words, they don't swing their arms excessively in front of their body.

Wasted motion in the arms is just as bad as an improper/inefficient stride in the legs. A few arm carriage don'ts include the following:

- Don't carry your arms too high—it will make your stride shorter than it should be and might result in tightness in your back.
- Don't carry your arms too low—your body will lean too far forward or in a side-to-side motion due to improper balance.

- Don't swing your elbows out too wide, as this too will result in throwing your balance off and negatively affecting your stride.
- Don't swing your arms too far inward, because too much inward swing can increase your chances of incurring hip injuries.

Posture

One of the biggest mistakes of many beginners is that they employ poor body posture when they run. Unless you're racing the 200 meters or shorter, don't lean forward. Doing so places great stress on your back and knees.

Proper posture begins with the correct body angle. To get a sense of this body angle, stand up straight against a wall. Your chest should be up but not out, your shoulders should be relaxed, and your buttocks should be pushed firmly back. This is the posture in which you should run. It will allow for correct breathing, will prevent you from leaning over and placing too much stress on your knees, lower legs, and back, and will help you to lengthen your stride and make knee lift easier. Finally, it will also help you to have a more efficient footstrike.

In thinking about your posture as you run, you should consider where your hips are when your foot hits the ground. Some people have suggested that your foot should be under the center of gravity of your body when it strikes the ground. A line from your head through your hips should end up at your foot. Keep your head fairly straight and look ahead. Turns to the side should be done carefully and usually mostly from the neck up to avoid twisting your body and making you unstable in your forward progression.

Nike cofounder Bill Bowerman, in his coaching days at the University of Oregon, advised his runners to run tall. This sums up the style of many of the recent and current greats in long-distance running. You should run standing up fairly straight, not leaning forward, twisted to one side, or tilting backwards. Look ahead at where you are going, and don't stare at your feet or the ground.

As you are running, also be careful that you don't stick your chest out, as doing so increases tightness and tension in all the muscles in your back and neck. Your shoulders should be relaxed. Sometimes, as you're able to build up time and mileage, your back may tighten up, usually because you're becoming tense. Therefore, even as you focus on good posture, remember to relax. You wan to run standing up straight but comfortably so.

The Mechanics of Running Hills

Because going up and down hills requires different mechanics than running on more level ground, some of the same mechanics that will benefit a long-distance runner are also those that will fail you in negotiating hills successfully. One of the few good things about hills is that they will force you to use muscles you don't normally use. In that respect, hills are excellent.

Running Uphill

While you won't be able to maintain the same speed running uphill as you do on the flats, try to maintain the same effort level. Move your arms a bit more to assist your legs. Imagine that you are cranking your way up or pulling yourself up the hill. Shorten your stride, lift your knees a bit, lean slightly into the hill, and power on up.

Running Downhill

One of the best things about coming downhill is that you can use gravity to your advantage. However, few people know how to really negotiate the downhill side effectively without losing control or slowing down. While your natural tendency is to lean back when going down hill, you should instead lean forward slightly to maintain a posture in relation to the ground as if you were running on the flats. Try to keep your footstrike light so as not to "grind" your heels into the hill as a braking mechanism. Use slight upper body positioning to make speed and body balance adjustments.

Runners with little prior experience with downhill running should be careful. The biggest risk of injury is to your knees. Your quadriceps do the bulk of the braking and can be overworked without you being aware of it.

If you are racing, then you may lean forward a bit and fly down the hill in a short race, but certainly be more careful in training. In fact, many runners who use hills as part of their advanced training will walk or lightly jog down the hill to recover before charging up again. This is a good way to rest and recover while avoiding the excessive knee stress that downhill running can cause.

Runner's Recap

As you develop proper running technique, remember the essentials of running mechanics. First, your posture should be guided by focusing on standing erect and imagining a cord coming out of the center and top of your head that gently pulls you straight up. Use your neck muscles to keep your head looking forward, not buried in your chest nor cocked back. Additionally, as you run, keep your face relaxed by letting your jaw drop and your cheeks "flap," and keep your eyes looking about ten to twenty feet ahead of you.

Concentrating on your body while running, pull up with your abdominal muscles and focus on running tall with your torso perpendicular to the running surface and your hips directly under your upper body. Let your shoulders hang relaxed and low, not drawn up toward your ears. Hold your arms close to your body, bending them at ninety-degree angles and keeping them near-parallel to the ground as they swing counter to your legs. At the same time, hold your hands in a loose fist, with the thumbs up and the palms facing each other.

With a light, efficient, short stride, each foot should land directly under the center of your body weight, not out in front of you. You should land lightly on your heel or ball (mid-foot), roll forward onto the ball of your foot, then push off with the balls of your feet and toes in a smooth, fluid, and relatively quiet motion.

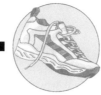

CHAPTER 5
Time to Get Going!

You're motivated, you're conscientious, you're equipped, and you have learned about proper mechanics. So, are you ready to go running? Or are you wondering where you should begin? Read on to determine what you need to do and how you are doing if this is your first time running.

Starting Out

Even if you've never run a step in your life, the training schedule included for you on page 51 will enable you to become a runner in a matter of a few short weeks. Where you choose to begin this schedule depends upon your current fitness level. If you're just getting into a cardiovascular exercise program, start at the beginning of Week #1 with brisk walking and proceed through the schedule as indicated. For individuals who presently are quite active (who, at a minimum, can easily walk at a brisk pace and/or jog nonstop for two minutes), begin following the schedule at Week #7.

To minimize your chances of incurring an injury, be patient and stick to the schedule. By all means, avoid the urge to do more than is specified. During the early weeks of the schedule, feel free to break up the cumulative minutes indicated for running into smaller segments if you feel it necessary. There's no problem in modifying the schedule to fit into your busy lifestyle so long as you keep the sequence of runs the same. For example, if Sunday is not a good day for you to run, the goal time/mileage indicated on that day can be shifted to another day of the week, as long as the sequence for the remainder of runs during the week is also shifted.

The pace of your running should be an aerobic level (meaning the ability to breathe easily without pushing yourself). In other words, you should be running very relaxed and comfortably. You should be able to talk in complete sentences without gasping for air. If you find yourself "huffing and puffing," you are probably running too fast and need to slow down your pace.

In the beginning, the key to success and evaluating your progress should be based on the *cumulative minutes* you are able to run without stopping rather than on the pace at which you run. With consistent training over a period of weeks, your running form will become more refined and efficient. This, in itself, often translates into a faster pace without the need to overload your present musculoskeletal system. Consider running for cumulative time rather than running the same measured route day after day. By doing so you will stay motivated and thus avoid burnout.

BEGINNER RUN/WALK SCHEDULE

WEEK #	SUN.	MON.	TUE.	WED.	THUR.	FRI.	SAT.	TOTAL
1	W-8	Rest	W-10	Rest	W-11	Rest	W-8	W-37
2	W-12	Rest	W-14	Rest	W-16	Rest	W-10	W-52
3	W-18	Rest	W-20	Rest	W-22	Rest	W-12	W-72
4	W-24	Rest	W-26	Rest	W-28	Rest	W-12	W-90
5	W-30	Rest	W-30	Rest	W-30	Rest	W-30	W-120
6	W-20	Rest	W-20	Rest	W-26	Rest	W-20	W-86 Light Week
7	R-2 W-28	Rest	R-3 W-27	Rest	R-4 W-26	Rest	W-30	R-9 W-81
8	R-5 W-25	Rest	R-6 W-24	Rest	R-8 W-22	Rest	R-6 W-24	R-25 W-95
9	R-10 W-20	Rest	R-11 W-19	Rest	R-12 W-18	Rest	R-8 W-22	R-41 W-79
10	R-14 W-16	Rest	R-16 W-14	Rest	R-18 W-12	Rest	R-10 W-20	R-58 W-62
11	R-20 W-10	Rest	R-22 W-8	Rest	R-24 W-6	Rest	R-12 W-18	R-78 W-42
12	R-26 W-4	Rest	R-28 W-2	Rest	R-30	Rest	R-14 W-16	R-96 W-22
13	R-20	Rest	R-20 W-10	Rest	R-26 W-4	Rest	R-16 W-14	R-82 W-26 Light Week
14	R-30	Rest	R-25 W-5	Rest	R-30	Rest	R-18 W-12	R-103 W17
15	R-33	Rest	R-30	Rest	R-30	Rest	R-20 W-10	R-113 W-10
16	R-36	Rest	R-30	Rest	R-30	Rest	R-20 W-10	R-116 W-10
17	R-39	Rest	R-30	Rest	R-30	Rest	R-30	R-129
18	R-20 W-10	Rest	R-20 W-10	Rest	R-26 W-4	Rest	R-20 W-10	R-86 W-34 Light Week

W = Walk; R = Run; Numbers = minutes of exercise

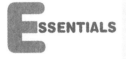
ESSENTIALS

Even if your goal is to run, don't ever be ashamed to walk. In fact, the first sections of the beginner schedule feature a mixture of walking and running. If you are unable to run the specified goal time/mileage on the schedule at the present time for whatever reason (aches, pain, fatigue, etc.), then by all means, walk the distance.

Learning How to Run

Despite the fact that you may be a few pounds over your ideal weight or even if you haven't exercised in years, if you can walk for fifteen or twenty minutes, this schedule can make you a runner. It can also take you to your first 5K in eighteen weeks!

When starting out, have fun, and don't give in to the desire to do too much too soon or worse, quit before you reap the benefits that running can provide you. Be patient with yourself and consistent in your workout. In short, enjoy the process but don't overdo it. Happiness in running comes from the journey, not the final destination.

Tips Before You Begin

Before you head out the door, review the following tips. Even though running is a simple activity, you need to be mindful of what you're doing at all times in order to maximize its benefits and your enjoyment.

Be Aware of Road Slants

Runners should pay attention to camber, or road slants, regardless of whether or not they have hip or knee problems, for frequent running on pitched/slanted surfaces increases your chances of incurring injury. If your knees or hips are prone to soreness, you should pay special attention to the camber—the slightly arched shape of the surface of the road or trail—and try to run on the flattest portion. This will reduce the angular stress that may make any injury problem a more serious one.

FACTS

The shortest distance between two points is a straight line. In training, it is fine to hug the wide lines. But when you are running in a road race or timed event, look for and run the shortest official course, especially on curves and turns. Hugging the outside border of the road can add mileage and time to your performance.

Stay Hydrated

For hot, humid days and for runs over half an hour, it is very important that you drink fluids every twenty-five to thirty minutes. Above all, don't wait until you're thirsty to start taking in fluids. Before setting out, drink eight ounces of water and hydrate regularly during your run. For runs lasting an hour or longer, it is important to also consume sports drinks such as Gatorade or Powerade.

To have more fluids available to you during your longer runs, there are a couple of options available to you. You can carry cool fluids with you (check out your options at your running supply or outdoor specialty stores). However, many people don't like carrying this added equipment while training. Additionally, you should avoid carrying fluid containers in your hands, as this throws off your form and also causes upper body fatigue.

ALERT

It's important to stay well-hydrated and drink a lot of fluids. But keep in mind one of the side effects of consuming so many fluids is more frequent trips to the bathroom. Therefore, be sure to use the bathroom before running, especially if you are a morning runner.

You can also plan your route so that you are able to stop at water fountains along the way. Another good idea is to stash bottled water and sports drinks along your course in advance. Lots of runners do this without too much difficulty, and it alleviates the problem described above of having to carry fluids with you. Doing so also offers the psychological advantage of breaking up the run mentally, since you can set yourself the goal of running from one fluid stop to the next.

Mind the Seasons

Certainly, one of the great things about running is that it is a year-round sport. You can run through every season as long as you adequately hydrate and dress appropriately. Dress warm enough in winter and cool enough in summer.

Be especially careful on extremely hot or cold days. You should always try to avoid running in extreme heat and extreme cold. If you really must run in such conditions, bring plenty of water with you or place water along the course of your run and consider shortening your workout for that day. There will be more tips about running in hot and cold weather in Chapter 9.

Minimize Risks

Running, like many other sports, poses its own set of potential problems, including dangers on the trail and the risk of injury. One of the most important things you can do is be aware of your surroundings. Keep your head up and your eyes focused ahead of you rather than down at your feet. If you run in the dark, make yourself visible to others with reflective clothing, decals, or tape. Carry a small flashlight so you can see where or what you are landing on. Let someone know where you are going, what time you left, and when you expect to return.

On a dirt trail, watch out for roots and rocks. Avoid running alone in areas that bears and mountain lions call home. For safety reasons, women should consider finding companions to accompany them when running in unpopulated areas. Dogs and human companions can be fun additions to running, and they provide security against some undesired interactions.

Don't overdo it, especially in the beginning. One of the negative effects of running excessive mileage or too frequently (for example, not scheduling regular rest days) is the possibility of incurring injury. Injuries to the knee, hip, and Achilles tendon, in particular, can often be attributed to overtraining. Listen to your body and don't make comparisons between your training program and the workouts/mileage totals of other runners.

Different degrees of pain after a workout may include soreness (a light, achy feeling); aches (continuous dull throbbing); and pains (acute and sharp hurting). If soreness or aches don't diminish, take some time off from running. If the pain increases, stay off the injury, apply RICE (rest, ice, compress, elevation), and take a pain reliever. If the pain doesn't subside in a few days, see a doctor.

Beginning Your Running Program

Remember that the safest and most enjoyable approach is to build your abilities up incrementally. By following the suggestions and schedules in this book, you will find your abilities as a runner increase safely and steadily.

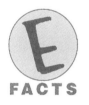

"I've been running since I was in my thirties, and had never broken the barrier from a few minutes to long distance. Until Art Liberman put me on a training program—and it worked. Beginning with twelve minutes, I am now able to run ninety-plus minutes non-stop."

—Margo Painter, Pensacola, FL

Building a Base

Without question, the most important area one should focus on prior to beginning any running program is safely and slowly building one's mileage. You should eventually be running four to five days a week with minimum mileage totals of twenty to twenty-five miles per week in anticipation of entering races longer than 10K (6.2 miles). You should not introduce advanced running techniques such as speed work, hill repeats, etc., into your training schedule until you're ready. At that point, longer runs and weekly mileage can be added in small increments.

Going to the Next Level

The mileage buildup schedule can be used to prepare the beginner/novice to run a ten-mile race (this is assuming that you have either completed the walk/run schedule and/or can run four miles prior to picking up this book). If you already have some running experience and wish to enter races longer than ten miles (such as the half-marathon and marathon) in the near future, put your current training on hold as you complete the last couple of weeks of this schedule.

Please also keep in mind that prior to your target race, include a taper period of one to two weeks where you reduce your mileage totals 35 to 40 percent. By doing so, you will be well rested and ready to perform optimally. Also keep in mind that the walk/run schedule can be used to "set the stage," so to speak, to prepare true beginners to complete (not race competitively) their first 5K.

The 10 Percent Rule

Do not increase either your weekly mileage or long-run mileage by more than 10 percent a week. Doing so greatly increases the chances of incurring an injury, thereby delaying or stopping your training all together. Refer to Chapter 12 for additional information. Many running injuries can be attributed to runners not following this simple but extremely important premise.

MILEAGE BUILDUP SCHEDULE

WEEK #	SUN.	MON.	TUE.	WED.	THUR.	FRI.	SAT.	TOTAL
1	4	Rest	3	Rest	4	Rest	3	14
2	4	Rest	4	Rest	4	Rest	3	15
3	5	Rest	4	Rest	4	Rest	3	16
4	3	Rest	3	Rest	3	Rest	3	12 LIGHT WEEK
5	5	Rest	4	Rest	4	Rest	4	17
6	6	Rest	4	Rest	4	Rest	4	18
7	6	Rest	4	Rest	5	Rest	4	19
8	3	Rest	4	Rest	3	Rest	3	13 LIGHT WEEK
9	7	Rest	4	Rest	5	Rest	4	20
10	7	Rest	5	Rest	5	Rest	4	21
11	8	Rest	5	Rest	5	Rest	4	22
12	4	Rest	3	Rest	4	Rest	4	15 LIGHT WEEK
13	8	Rest	5	Rest	6	Rest	4	23
14	9	Rest	5	Rest	6	Rest	4	24
15	9	Rest	6	Rest	6	Rest	4	25
16	5	Rest	4	Rest	4	Rest	4	17 LIGHT WEEK
17	10	Rest	6	Rest	6	Rest	4	26
18	10	Rest	6	Rest	7	Rest	4	27
19	6	Rest	4	Rest	5	Rest	4	19 LIGHT WEEK

*NUMBERS REFER TO MINUTES OF RUNNING

ADVANCED MILEAGE BUILDUP SCHEDULE

WEEK #	SUN.	MON.	TUE.	WED.	THUR.	FRI.	SAT.	TOTAL
1	4	Rest	3	Rest	4	Rest	3	14
2	4	Rest	4	Rest	4	Rest	3	15
3	5	Rest	4	Rest	4	Rest	3	16
4	3	Rest	3	Rest	3	Rest	3	12 Light Week
5	5	Rest	3	3	3	Rest	3	17
6	6	Rest	3	3	3	Rest	3	18
7	6	Rest	3	4	3	Rest	4	20
8	3	Rest	4	Rest	3	Rest	3	13 Light Week
9	7	Rest	3	5	4	Rest	3	22
10	7	Rest	4	5	4	Rest	4	24
11	8	Rest	4	6	4	Rest	4	26
12	4	Rest	3	Rest	4	Rest	4	15 Light Week
13	8	Rest	5	6	5	Rest	4	28
14	9	Rest	5	5	6	Rest	4	29
15	9	Rest	5	7	6	Rest	5	32
16	5	Rest	4	Rest	4	Rest	4	17 Light Week
17	10	Rest	6	8	6	Rest	4	34
18	10	Rest	6	8	7	Rest	4	35
19	6	Rest	4	Rest	5	Rest	4	19 Light Week

Beginning Runner's Mistakes

Watch out for common mistakes that beginning runners often make. These may include:

- **Focusing on speed:** Try to focus on increasing your duration rather than speed as a means of evaluating your progress.
- **Doing too much too soon:** Increasing mileage as a result of overenthusiasm often leads to the most common beginner running injury—shin splints.
- **Not listening to your body:** If excessively sore or fatigued, either walk or take an extra day off.
- **Using old running shoes or shoes not designed specifically for running:** Run in shoes that are biomechanically appropriate to your body's running needs.
- **Training with the wrong people:** Run with others who are at your ability level, not with those who run either much faster or slower than you.
- **Trying to emulate other people's running styles:** Use the proper form when you run to avoid discomfort or injury.

A More Advanced Schedule

When you have completed your choice of either buildup schedule, you will have developed a base from which you may now consider training for race distances longer than ten miles. The advanced mileage buildup schedule features five days of training (on most weeks) and more weekly mileage than the previous mileage buildup schedule.

So how do you decide which schedule to choose? Some readers of this book will already be at or above the level of the basic buildup schedule and will want other mileage buildup options. These runners have the time and desire to train five days a week. If this describes you, make sure you are up to it and can comfortably train at this level. Don't push yourself too hard by selecting a schedule that does not yet match your present level of conditioning.

At the conclusion of Week #19 of either schedule, assuming that you've made it through the mileage buildup stage without injury, you are now ready to proceed to new training goals. These might include incorporating more advanced training techniques (such as speed work) and/or training for longer races such as the half-marathon and marathon.

Staying Motivated

As you progress through your training schedule, you might feel discouraged or unmotivated at points. You can stay motivated by doing the following:

- Choose some goals that you'd like to accomplish (enter a local 5K, lose a few pounds, tone up your leg muscles, and so on).
- Plan out your week well in advance to allow time to train or a specific time of the day to fit in your running and don't let others change your plans.
- Be patient and persistent, realizing that it will take some time to be able to run twenty to thirty minutes non-stop.
- Visualize the way you hope to look a few months from now and then go for it!

CHAPTER 6

Ready for Racing: The 5K

The 5K offers all runners an array of challenges. Experienced runners may wish to improve their time from a previous race, whereas beginning runners might simply hope to finish the event. Regardless of your motivation, the 5K is a goal that can be accomplished after just a few short weeks of training.

5K Basics

The 5K in actuality is only 3.1 miles. By the time you complete the first training schedule, you'll be able to at least finish a 5K without months of intense preparation, even if you have to walk for part or all of it.

You will find that 5K events are a lot of fun. The races are usually well-organized and are often supported by corporate sponsors, area businesses, a running club, or perhaps a local booster organization. These races are like little running fairs. Participants sometimes receive T-shirts, samples of running foods like Power Bars, gel energy supplements, fruit, honey sticks, and other running products, as well as a wealth of information about other races close to the locale where you are running.

Also attendant at many 5Ks are small local running specialty stores who feature wares such as new running shoes, running apparel, and other running-related accessories. It is not uncommon for people to have some fun indulging in a little shopping either just before or just after the race.

Of course, you'll also see a lot of other runners at 5K events. They come alone, in pairs, or in groups, all from diverse backgrounds. Buddies, girlfriends, couples, and families all attend, and they all love running, as well as socializing with fellow runners.

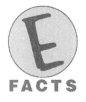

FACTS

The larger 5K races across the country typically include at least one vendor of running gear. These are great venues to find sales on the basics: shorts, socks, and even shoes. Reward yourself for competing in the event by supplementing your running wardrobe before you go home!

Race Strategy and Goal Setting

Goal setting is indeed important. Not only does it keep your training in focus, but it makes competing in races both fun and challenging. In the weeks prior to the race, think about three goals you'd be interested in accomplishing: an easily obtainable goal, a realistic yet moderately challenging goal, and an ultimate goal. Be realistic. For example, if you don't possess the genetic gift to run a sub sixteen-minute 5K, don't set that as your ultimate goal.

Some 5K goals might include completing the entire event running, improving your time by thirty seconds to a full minute or coming in under a specific time. By making sure these goals are realistic, you will avoid being disappointed when you could be satisfied or even thrilled with your performance. Above all, it's important to keep everything in perspective. Sure, you would have loved to run a faster time; still, be thankful that you are healthy and are able to walk, let alone run.

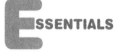

SSENTIALS

Sure, races are competitive. Sure, you want to do your best. But remember that one of the great things about running is that you're mostly competing with yourself. So put things in perspective, give yourself an achievable goal, and keep the fun in the 5K.

The Week Before Your 5K

There is no workout you can do in the one week prior to your 5K that will enhance your performance. Therefore, make the final week prior to the big race an easy one with light workouts (continue to follow either of the mileage buildup charts in Chapter 5). Make one of the two days prior to the event a complete leg-rest day.

Don't break with your training schedule or try anything radically different the week before your race, either. For example, one of the most frequent mistakes that comes back to haunt the unknowing runner, whether it be in a short event or a marathon, is to run in new shoes purchased the day before the race. It takes at least a few training runs for new shoes to get broken in. Wearing new shoes even a few days before the race could cause a variety of problems, such as blisters and foot discomfort, which can affect your performance in the race.

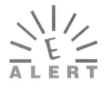

Don't try anything radically new or different in the weeks before your 5K. Don't try a new diet, don't try new shoes. Taper your mileage at an easy pace, get adequate rest, and prepare yourself mentally for the big day.

What to Eat and Drink

Nutrition principles dictate that you should always stay well hydrated, whether you are exercising or not. In particular, drink ample fluids in the days prior to competition, regardless of the event distance or race day environmental conditions.

For workouts and races that last an hour or less, water taken every twenty-five to thirty minutes is all that is needed to stay well-hydrated. Although sports drinks do play an important role during runs lasting an hour and longer (which we will address later in Chapters 11 and 16), they won't necessarily give you a performance edge for shorter workouts and events such as the 5K. Consuming sports drinks can be especially helpful when training in hot and humid conditions as they refuel your body's electrolyte stores.

Eating Before Race Day

Carbohydrate-loading and eating in general is one of the great aspects of running, whether it be to fuel your body for training runs or road races. However, you really don't need to load up too much on carbohydrates the day or two before a 5K, not in the same way that one needs to do for a marathon.

Don't stuff yourself thinking you're only going to burn it off the next day. And don't eat new things that you've not experimented with during your training. Many a runner has rued the time that he or she decided to have some exotic or unfamiliar foods the day before a race. Eat something you know will agree with you. Otherwise, regardless of your pace, the consequences of poor nutritional choices could be discomforting and perhaps even embarrassing.

In summary, your evening meal the day before the race should consist of well-balanced but simple foods that you know will cause no digestive troubles. A mix of 65 percent carbohydrates, 20 percent protein, and 15 percent fat is optimal. Avoid foods that are high in salt or fat and that are fried. You will also want to limit your intake of foods with high roughage content, such as salads, vegetables, and cereals.

ESSENTIALS   If you're like most runners, you live for your next meal. Well, plan your eating extravagances for the night after the 5K. Leading up to the event, be mindful of any unnecessary fat, sugar, or other nutritional "bombs" that might put you in the Port-a-John instead of on the starting line the day of the race.

Drinking Before Race Day

As is continually stressed throughout this book, drink a lot of water. If you enjoy beverages that contain caffeine such as coffee or tea, be aware that drinking these in the late afternoon or evening may make it difficult for you to fall asleep easily, especially if you've got pre-race jitters. Additionally, both caffeine as well as alcoholic beverages are diuretics that can contribute to dehydration.

Eating on Race Day

Equally important is your decision regarding what to eat on race day. If the race is set for early in the morning, as most 5Ks are, you may wish to bypass breakfast and just stick with water. If you choose to eat a light snack (this could be a banana, slice of toast, bagel, or energy bar), be sure that it is consumed at least one hour before the start of the race.

Events held during the late morning, mid-afternoon, or evening are more difficult to plan for nutritionally. One has to be much more careful regarding food selection when the run will be fast paced. While you certainly don't want to go hungry in the hours prior to a race or a fast-paced workout, you don't want to eat foods that will cause stomach cramps or digestive problems.

Light healthy snacks are your best approach for late morning and early afternoon races. If the race will be held in the evening, eat a healthy and satisfying breakfast along with a sensible but light lunch (avoid high-fat and fried foods). Foods such as a piece of fruit or a handful of pretzels are great snack choices later in the afternoon. In short, the best way to determine what foods and fluids will work best for you whether it be during training runs or races is by experimenting with these in practice.

Get a Good Night's Sleep

Try to go to bed early the night prior to the race so that you will be well rested for the event. This will also make waking up to the alarm a bit easier than normal. Above all, you won't be rushed or, worse, oversleep and miss the race. Wake up early enough to eat, make a visit to the bathroom, and take care of anything you feel the need to do so as not to feel rushed. If you want to do your best in a 5K, it's important to be rested and ready.

Packing for the Race

Lay out everything you need (apparel, shoes, etc.) the evening before the race so that you will save yourself time, stress, and aggravation in the morning. You won't want to be halfway there and realize you forgot something, especially if you have to help others get ready to go with you. It's important that you have everything you need taken care of in plenty of time.

ALERT

Don't overpack when going to a race. Between the freebies you're given at the race and the goods you'll want to buy, you may have a lot to carry. If you're walking to the race, take a small bag that can be checked at the start. If you drive to the race, you can put your items in your car.

Physical Preparation

Listen to your body. As mentioned above, there are no workouts the week prior to the 5K or any race distance event that will enhance your preparedness for the race. A general rule of thumb is "less is best." The physiological effects of training don't kick in for a week to ten days, so the workout today will not immediately enhance your levels of performance.

Remember also not to try anything new the week prior to or during your 5K. There are so many heartbreaking stories of runners who tried something new in the week prior to a race, only to injure themselves and end up not being able to participate in the event at all. Don't let that happen to you.

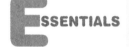

ESSENTIALS

The following are some 5K pre-race reminders:

- Preregister for the event to save time and money.
- Remember the race will begin on time and regardless of almost any weather conditions (except perhaps lightening storms).
- Arrive at the race site early.

Psychological Issues and Concerns

Remember that it is normal to be tense or nervous prior to a road race of any distance. Even the most seasoned runners experience these feelings. Stay away from participants who are excessively stressed out or negative. Don't let these individuals negatively affect your state of mind.

During the Race

As you are running the 5K, it's easy to get caught up in the excitement of it all. Just be sure that you keep the following essential guidelines in mind to ensure you have the best experience possible.

The Start

While runners are generally very honest people, this sometimes does not hold true when they are asked to line up for the start of the race according to their anticipated pace. Unfortunately, too many slower runners line up in front of the faster runners. In addition to this not being fair, in a large race the slower runners can actually create problems (as people tend to be pushed down or slip and fall). Please be courteous! Take a deep breath and know that you are going to have fun, stay relaxed, and achieve your goals.

Pacing and Staying Relaxed

Running the appropriate pace for your ability level is crucial for all distances, from sprints to the marathon, to enhance your chances of performing optimally and running your fastest possible race. It is so easy to start the race running much faster than you should. Your pace during the first mile may feel effortless due to the adrenaline rush and excitement of the event. But this can cause you to burn out by the second or third mile.

Running each mile at the same pace has been proven to be the best approach to turning in your best race time. If it feels like you're really overextending yourself, you probably are. Taper back a bit and see if you feel like catching some folks at the end. You'll enjoy finishing strong.

Another way to avoid draining your energy too quickly is to remember to stay loose and relaxed. Be sure to shake out your arms and shoulders occasionally throughout the race to avoid upper body muscle tightness. This will contribute to a more comfortable run.

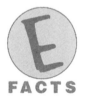

FACTS

Chances are you'll run faster in a race than you do during your training runs, even if it's not your goal to go faster. The rush of the crowd and the fact that it's a race contribute to the excitement, which usually translates into a faster pace.

Water Stops and Supplements

All races have water stops, at which eager volunteers hold out cups of water for you to take as you pass. Mastering the art of drinking while you're running takes some time. But the only way to do it is to, well, do it. So give it a try. If you're not too successful and get most of the water on your face or shirt, oh well. What you don't want to do is inhale the water and end up choking. So if it's easier and more comfortable for you, just slow down to a walk for a few steps while you drink.

If it's a really hot day, you can also pour water over your head, on your neck, chest, and hands. As for supplements like energy gels or a sports beverage, you don't really need them in a 5K.

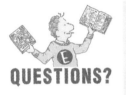

QUESTIONS?

What if you get injured during the race?
If you feel a significant increase in pain as you continue to run, seriously consider dropping out of the race. No race is worth the risk of hurting yourself by continuing to run and causing a minor injury to turn into a major setback.

After the Race

Congratulations, you did it! Savor the excitement of finishing, no matter where you came in. Then, after crossing the line, get something to drink. Within a few minutes of finishing, do a five- to ten-minute cool-down jog to begin the recovery process. Stretch thoroughly immediately afterwards. Doing so will keep muscle soreness to a minimum over the next day or two. And, of course, chat about the race with your fellow runners.

When you get home, look at the flyers you collected at the race to think about when and where you will run your next 5K (or maybe an even longer race). If you're like most runners, you'll be hooked on the great feeling of having successfully competed in the race.

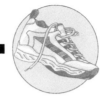

CHAPTER 7

Don't Forget to Stretch

Stretching is an extremely important part of running. Stretching keeps your muscles from cramping and reduces the possibility of injury. It helps to lengthen your muscles and improve your flexibility. In the end, it will improve and lengthen stride and increase your overall speed and stamina. However, if you stretch incorrectly or spottily, you may end up doing more harm than good.

Stretching Before the Run

One of the greatest misconceptions about running is that one must stretch beforehand. In fact, the opposite is the case; you should stretch after a workout. If you really feel you should stretch because you want to loosen up or warm up your muscles before the serious work, jog or walk for five or ten minutes and then stretch. The best thing to do is to start your run very slowly, then ease into a training pace five to ten minutes later. The idea is not to stretch a cold muscle. If you're planning to do a speed workout or race, jog for about a mile, stretch, then do striders, and do the speed workout or race. Warm-up procedures are discussed in depth in Chapter 11.

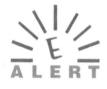

Before stretching, you need to warm those muscles up. Don't stretch past the point of slight discomfort. If your muscles are still cold, don't try to stretch them like a rubber band, especially if you haven't run in a while.

Stretching after the Run

It's very important to remember that you need to stretch after the run. A workout isn't over until, as part of your cool-down period, you stretch thoroughly immediately following the run. You need to make sure you establish the good work habits of successful runners, and the stretching period after the run is as important as the run itself.

View stretching as a part of your overall workout. It should be just as natural and routine as jogging to warm up before an event. This is because your legs will be most receptive to the benefits of stretching *immediately* after you run. Stretching thirty to forty minutes later when your muscles have cooled down increases your chances of causing injury. Your muscles are fatigued and tight after a run, especially a long or fast-paced one, and stretching can help to alleviate soreness later.

In short, stretch gently and slowly while your muscles are still warm. One final rule: No bouncing when you stretch. This is called ballistic stretching, and it can cause injuries!

Stretching Fundamentals

Whenever you stretch, remember the objectives of stretching, which are to improve flexibility, strengthen and lengthen your muscles so they can perform optimally, prevent injuries, and enhance circulation. When you integrate stretching into your overall workout routine, you'll be amazed by how much better you'll feel all over.

How to Stretch Properly

Have you ever seen someone go about stretching haphazardly? They throw their foot onto a fence post or railing, awkwardly bend toward it, bounce a few times, try to grab their foot a couple of times, then heave their foot back down and start with the other one. Common sense says there's something wrong with this all-too-common sight, and there is.

To be effective, stretching needs to be slow, gentle, and focused. Concentrate on the muscles or muscle groups you're working on and breathe naturally and regularly (no holding your breath). Inhale as you set up the stretch, exhale as you lean into the stretch, moving slowly and lightly to extend the muscle to its greatest point of extension. Stop when you feel mild tension and hold the stretch for thirty to sixty seconds. At the end of that time, inhale out of the stretch as gently as you went into it.

Patience Is a Virtue

Even if you presently have poor flexibility, a regular stretching program will greatly improve your range of motion. The keys are to be both patient and consistent. Your stretching should not cause pain, although it may feel a bit uncomfortable at first or even awkward when extending a muscle to the far end of its present range of motion.

You can also supplement your stretching with exercises that strengthen your muscles to further support your joints and skeleton. For example, strengthening your abdominals by doing crunches and situps correctly, or building up your arms and shoulders using free weights or machines such as Nautilus or Cybex, are ways you can benefit your overall health and improve your running. These techniques are covered in Chapter 8.

ESSENTIALS

Static stretch basics:

- Stretch the muscle to the point of its greatest range of motion, but don't overextend.
- Never bounce when stretching; rather, hold the stretch for thirty to sixty seconds.
- Stretch all the major leg muscle groups.
- Stretch uniformly (after stretching one leg, stretch the other).
- Don't overstretch an injured area as this may cause additional damage.

The Best Stretches for Runners

The stretches described here will benefit the major muscles in your legs—those that support your shins, thighs, ankles, knees, hips, and buttocks.

Stretching the Hamstring

Your hamstrings are located in the backs of your thighs. When they're too tight, you may experience lower back pain. To stretch them out, stand with your feet shoulder-width apart and pointing straight ahead. Start to bend over at the waist, moving your hands toward your feet. Keep your knees slightly bent as you do this and only go as far down as it takes to feel a minimal tightness.

As you bend down, relax your neck and shoulders and slowly exhale. When you reach the slightly tight point, relax into it and hold for approximately thirty seconds. When the time is up, start straightening back up as you inhale. Move slowly and allow your head to roll up gently as well. When you're back in the standing position, exhale. Inhale as you begin to bend forward again.

Repeat this stretch three to five times. If you do this after every run, you'll notice improvements in your flexibility within a week. Soon you'll be able to reach your knees, then your ankles, and, yes, your toes!

Quadriceps, Knees, and Iliotibial Band

Until you develop the leg strength, you should do this stretch while holding on to or leaning against something for support. To stretch your right quads and IT band, support yourself with your right hand. Bend your right knee while grabbing your foot with your left hand. With your toes slightly pointed, gently bring your foot toward your buttocks as you exhale. Hold the stretch for about thirty seconds. Switch legs. Repeat until you've stretched both legs three to four times. You can work on improving your balance with this stretch, too, by steadying yourself on the leg you're standing on and removing your hand from the wall or railing.

FACTS

The quadriceps (quads) and iliotibial band (IT band) support the knees during exercise. Quads are the muscles in the front of your thigh; the IT band runs from your hip to your knee along the outside of your leg. The stronger these muscles are, the better they can support your knees.

The Lower Body All-Over Stretch

Stand with your feet shoulder-width apart and your toes pointing out slightly. Keeping your feet flat, start to lower yourself into a squat. Exhale. Your knees should be outside of your shoulders but over your big toes. Support yourself with your arms in front of you and between your legs, hands touching the floor (if possible). You may want to do this with your back against a wall for additional support.

When you're squatting, hold the stretch for about thirty seconds. Come up slowly, inhaling as you straighten. Repeat two to three times when you're first learning this stretch. As you get better, hold it for a bit longer and see if you can repeat it four to five times.

FACTS

The squat stretch is a great stretch for your lower back, ankles, Achilles tendons, shins, and groin. If you spend a lot of time sitting or standing, you'll come to love this stretch. However, if you're a beginner, it could be particularly tough—go easy!

Stretching the Hips

The hip flexor can help keep you flexible through the hips. Sitting with your legs crossed in front of you, use both arms to take the foot and knee of one leg and stretch them toward you, cradling your leg. Hold for about thirty seconds and switch legs. Repeat a few times with each leg.

A Simple, Effective Stretching Routine

Stretching is something runners tend to skip because they never got into the routine of doing it or they felt they were doing it incorrectly. To avoid being one of those runners, use this simple routine of four stretches that can be done in about ten minutes.

First, stretch out your hamstrings. Lying on your back with your legs extended, bend one leg and bring your knee up toward your chest. Use both hands to hold your leg into your chest. Grasp your leg as far down as you can, making it a goal to be able to grab your foot as you hold the stretch. Hold for approximately thirty seconds, switch legs, and work toward four to five repetitions, alternating legs.

Next, you will stretch your hips. Shift from lying down to sitting and do the hip flexor stretch described here.

After the hip flex, you will stretch your quadriceps. You will move from a sitting to a standing position. Lean against a wall or hold a firm rail for support. Then, follow the directions for stretching quadriceps described previously in this chapter.

Finally, you will stretch the Achilles tendon, calf, and IT band. Standing with your feet shoulder-width apart, lean forward with your hands out against a wall, tree, or rail so that your body is at a forty-five-degree angle. Bending your knees, bring one leg about one stride in toward the wall. Keep both feet flat on the ground. Lean into the stretch, feeling it in the back of your leg and through your ankle.

CHAPTER 8

Weight Training and Cross-Training

Weight training and cross-training, like stretching, can enhance your running by both improving your performance and reducing your chances of incurring injury. By increasing muscle mass you can improve abdominal, back, arm, and leg strength. How you train and what exercises you choose will have a great impact on your running success.

Weight Training Benefits

Whether you are young or old, heavy or lean, a long-distance runner or a sprinter, you will benefit from weight training, also known as strength training. The increase in lean muscle mass that results from strength training is key to overall strength and to your body's ability to burn calories. This is because muscle cells require more energy (and also burn more calories) than fat cells.

After the age of thirty, people's muscle mass gradually begins to diminish. As this occurs, people notice that they can no longer eat all that they used to without gaining body fat. You may weigh less at age forty-five than you did at thirty-five, but body composition testing might indicate that you are carrying more body fat than at a younger age. Incorporating strength training three times or so per week to one's personal schedule can slow this process considerably.

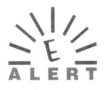

If you have any medical problems, such as heart disease, diabetes, or high blood pressure, or if you are over forty, see your doctor before beginning strength training. If you have carpal tunnel syndrome or any other upper extremity physical problem you should also consult your physician prior to beginning a strength training program.

Overall fitness requires more than just cardiovascular fitness. A balance of endurance, strength, and flexibility must be achieved. The most often recognized components of fitness include:

- Muscular fitness, strength, and endurance
- Flexibility
- Cardiovascular endurance
- Balanced nutrition
- Body composition

The last item, body composition, acts as a guide to how you are really doing. It is not a pure component of fitness. Although running is one of the best cardiovascular activities, besides strengthening a few specific muscles and rapidly burning a lot of calories, it does not fulfill many of the other criterions of overall fitness. That is why weight training is essential to your overall health.

Upper Body Benefits of Weight Training

A strong upper body enables a runner to maintain form late in a marathon or long run. Additionally, upper body strength reduces fatigue and stiffness in the arms, shoulders, and neck areas. Strong arms and shoulders are helpful in propelling a runner uphill. Finally, legs move only as fast as the arm swing. Thus, a runner with a strong upper body will run faster and more efficiently.

Leg Benefits of Weight Training

Running creates a muscular imbalance in the legs. Through running, one's hamstrings and calf muscles develop at a faster rate than the quadriceps and shins. Weight training helps address this imbalance. Additionally, strong quadriceps and hips help protect these areas from a variety of injuries. Strong legs also offer protection from the possibility of injury when running fast downhill.

Other Benefits of Weight Training

Weight training also helps protect bones. This is an important benefit, particularly for women, as decreased estrogen production causes bone demineralization, which, in turn, increases the risks of osteoporosis and stress fractures. The gentle pulling action of muscles on bone that happens during weight training facilitates bone regeneration.

Weight training may also help prevent life-threatening illnesses. Some studies show that strength training seems to reduce the risk factors for adult-onset diabetes as well as heart disease.

Upper Body Versus Lower Body

While many athletes train the entire body with equal intensity and will use heavy weights for their legs, heavy strength training for the legs is not necessarily vital or helpful for the long-distance runner. All of the elite athletes and advanced competitive runners use strength training (long-distance runners in particular, during their prime), emphasizing the upper body during their training. As some runners age, they find that more lower extremity exercises are helpful. Some of these runners have then generalized that if it is good for the aging athlete, it is good for the younger one too. That is not necessarily so.

Younger athletes aren't losing muscle by 5 to 20 percent; they are still in their prime. These runners are probably better off performing only a light lower extremity workout in combination with different running techniques to enhance their running speed, form, and strength. These techniques, discussed in greater depth in Chapter 11, include fartlek workouts, striders, hill repeats, tempo runs, and repeat intervals.

Marathon champion Bill Rogers, in his heyday, used dumbbells for upper body strength but did not perform strength training for his legs. Similarly, running legend Alberto Salazar, reportedly a recent convert to lower extremity strength training, also did not target this area in training while running his 120-plus mile weeks and winning marathons. Following their examples, go easy on the legs, using strength training cautiously with high repetitions and low weights while emphasizing upper body work.

Of course, there is value to gentle leg extensions, leg presses, leg curls, straight leg lifts, and (sometimes) gentle calf raises, as well as crunches. Just don't go overboard on the muscles that runners exercise the most.

More About the Main Muscles

Since you're going to be working muscles you might not have known you even had, the following is a brief anatomy lesson to help you both identify and appreciate your muscles. Knowing where the muscles are located and what they do enables you to understand what you're working out and why.

FIGURE 8-1:
Our muscles:
front view

FIGURE 8-2:
Our muscles:
back view

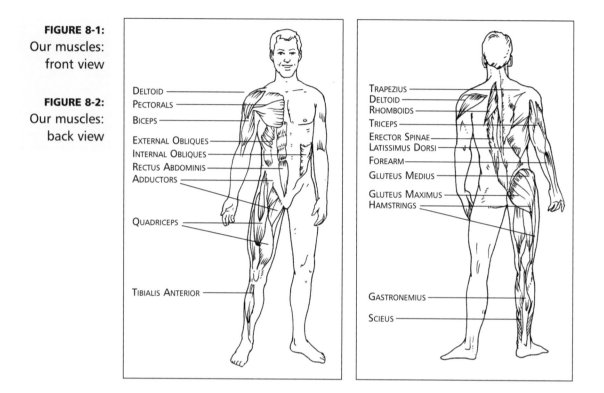

Front view labels: Deltoid, Pectorals, Biceps, External Obliques, Internal Obliques, Rectus Abdominis, Adductors, Quadriceps, Tibialis Anterior

Back view labels: Trapezius, Deltoid, Rhomboids, Triceps, Erector Spinae, Latissimus Dorsi, Forearm, Gluteus Medius, Gluteus Maximus, Hamstrings, Gastronemius, Scieus

Shoulders, Back, and Chest

A variety of muscles work together in your shoulders, back, and chest (see **FIGURES 8-1** and **8-2**). The muscles that traverse your chest below your breasts are called pectoralis but are commonly referred to as "pecs." Stretching along the tops of your arms near your shoulders are your deltoids. Nearby are your rotator cuffs, a group of four muscles under your shoulder that are used for carrying, catching, and throwing. The trapezius is a diamond-shaped muscle that runs across the shoulders, toward the neck and into the lower back.

In your back, you'll find the *erector spinae*, the muscles that run the length of the spine and that flex to straighten, bend, sit, stand, and lie down. Also running down your back is the *latissiumus dorsi*, a large muscle that goes from below your shoulder to your lower back. In the center of your back are triangular-shaped muscles, known as rhomboids, which keep the shoulder blades together and assist in proper posture.

Arms and Abs

The muscles of your arms and midsection are also important (see **FIGURES 8-1** and **8-2**). In your arms, the biceps are the muscles on the front of your arm, the ones you flex when someone asks to see how strong you are. The companion muscles to the biceps are the triceps. These are located on the back of your upper arm.

On the midsection, you will find your obliques and *rectus abdominis*. There are internal and external obliques that line both sides of your midsection and support the *rectus abdominis*. Meanwhile, *rectus abdominis* muscles extend from below the chest to just below the navel. They are more commonly referred to as "abs."

Hips, Butt, and Legs

Essential to runners, the major lower body muscles are the *gluteus maximus*, *gluteus medius*, and *gluteus minimus*, all of which are commonly called "gluts" (see **FIGURES 8-1** and **8-2**). Other lower body muscles include the hamstrings (a group of three muscles at the back of the thigh) and the quadriceps (a group of four muscles on the front of the thigh). You should also be aware of the *tibialis anterior*, a group of muscles that extends along your tibia (the bone that goes from your knee to your ankle, along the shin).

Practical Weight Training

Since this is a running book, the weight training exercises included here will be ones that you can do at home and that will still give you all the benefits described above. Although these exercises won't necessitate your going to the gym, if you want to take this training to the next level, go for it! Work with someone knowledgeable at the gym so you are using the appropriate amount of weight to work the muscles you want to target. And remember what was said about overworking your legs—it's not a good idea.

Types of Weights to Use

If you're starting as a complete beginner, the best weights to use are dumbbells, which you can buy at a sporting goods store. Dumbbells are convenient, portable, and not overwhelming. You can use them while watching television or talking on the phone. They come in various weights, and you'll need a few so you can use different ones to work different muscles. If the only upper body work you've done is lifting utensils to eat and drink, you'll probably want to start out with three-pound weights. You'll graduate to five pounds in a few weeks and may be ready to work with ten-pound weights in a few months.

You may also want to purchase weights for lower body work. A handy type of weight to use for leg strengthening is the kind that goes around your ankle and is adjusted with a Velcro strap. Again, be sure not to overdo it with leg exercises!

Using the Weights

There are two ways to hold your dumbbells: overhand and underhand. For the overhand grip, grab the dumbbell with your palm facing down and knuckles facing up. For the underhand grip, your palm should be facing up and your knuckles down.

There are two ways to stand as well. One is with your feet shoulder-width apart, head and shoulders level, back erect, and knees slightly bent. This is the standard "stand." The other position is bent over, feet shoulder-width apart, with one leg slightly extended. The idea is to work with a flat back and with your non-working arm resting on the same-side thigh.

How Many Reps?

When first beginning a strength training program, you should only perform one set of each exercise for the first couple of weeks, doing twelve to fifteen repetitions (reps) of an exercise. Don't feel overwhelmed and think you must increase the number of sets to reap strength training benefits. After this you may increase to two to three sets after one warm-up set. If you feel as if you could go well beyond fifteen to twenty reps, increase the weight on your next set or at your next session.

Upper Body Exercises

Your upper body workout should target the upper body muscles described above. Remember, for maximum results, use the appropriate weight (the weight at which you can do no more than twelve to fifteen reps).

Upper Body Biceps Curl and Triceps Kickback

From the standing position, arms at your side, hold the dumbbell with an underhand grip. With your elbow securely against your side, raise (curl) the dumbbell up and toward your chest as far as it will go, then control the weight as you bring your hand back down (see **FIGURE 8-3**). This is one repetition. Alternate arms after doing one set with one arm.

FIGURE 8-3:
Biceps curl

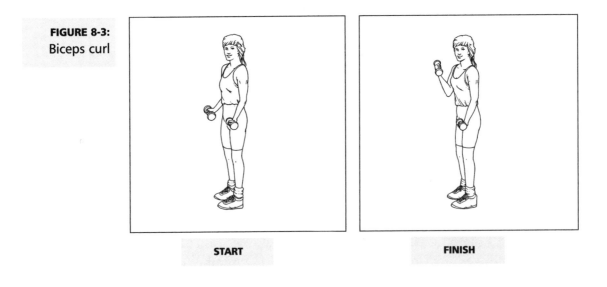

START   FINISH

FIGURE 8-4:
Bent-over
position

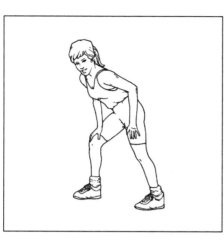

For the triceps kickback, use an overhand grip and, in the bent-over position (see **FIGURE 8-4**), extend the working arm straight behind you (kick it back) without hyperextending your arm (see **FIGURE 8-5**). Control the weight as you bend back toward your chest. This is one repetition.

FIGURE 8-5:
Triceps
kickback

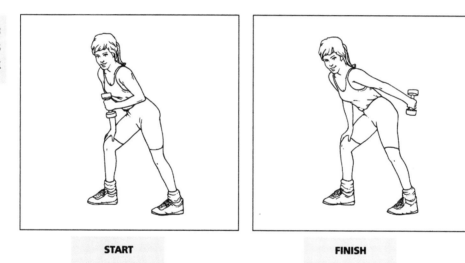

START   FINISH

Upper Body Front Raise

This exercise works your deltoids. In the standing position with the dumbbell in an overhand grip, let both arms rest in front of your body so that your palms are resting on your thighs. Then lift one arm straight up to shoulder height so that it's parallel to the floor (see **FIGURE 8-6**). Control the weight on the way back to the starting position for one repetition.

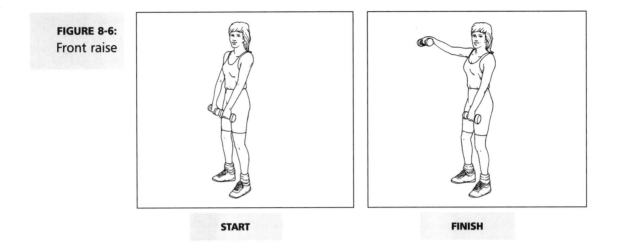

FIGURE 8-6:
Front raise

START   FINISH

Upper Body Shoulder Press

Standing with the dumbbells in an overhand grip, bend your arms so that the dumbbells are by your ears, palms facing away from your body. Extend your arm up and slightly in front of your head, then lower to the starting position for one rep (see **FIGURE 8-7**).

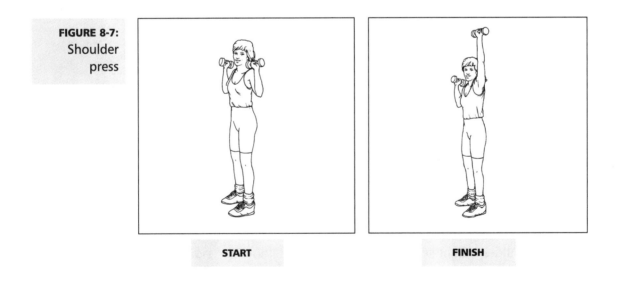

FIGURE 8-7:
Shoulder
press

START   FINISH

Upper Body Bent-Over Row

From the bent-over position, hold the dumbbell in an overhand grip and extend your arm toward the floor in a diagonal line from your shoulder. As if you were rowing a boat, bend your elbow and lift the dumbbell so that you use your back muscles as well as your arm muscles (see **FIGURE 8-8**). Pretend you're starting a lawnmower but with a smoother action. Return to the starting position for one rep.

FIGURE 8-8:
Bent-over
row

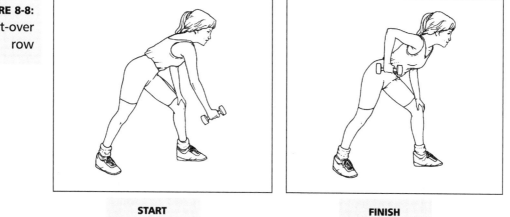

START   FINISH

Three Great Lower Body Exercises

These exercises will target your major lower body muscles. Keep in mind that as a runner, you don't want to overwork your legs, which get a workout every time you run.

Lunges

Stand with feet shoulder width apart, a dumbbell in each hand in the overhand grip. Step out with your right leg about one stride, landing on your heel and rolling your foot down flat against the floor. Bend both knees so that your right thigh is parallel to the floor. Your left thigh will be perpendicular to it, and your left heel will lift off the floor (see **FIGURE 8-9**). Your arms remain by your sides during the exercise. Return to the starting position by rolling off the ball of your right foot. Alternate legs as you do your reps.

FIGURE 8-9:
Lunge

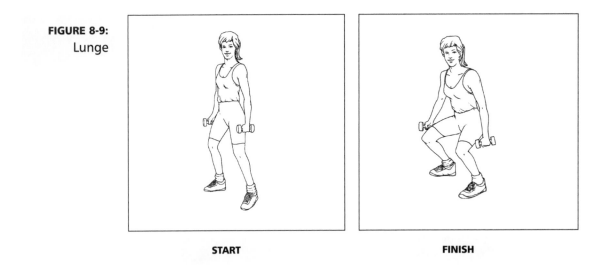

START   FINISH

Leg Extensions

Choose a chair with firm back support and in which, when you're sitting, your feet rest flat on the floor. Sitting in the chair, put the ankle weights on both feet. One leg at a time, squeeze with your thigh as you lift your leg until your knee is straight (see **FIGURE 8-10**). Control the descent. This is one rep.

FIGURE 8-10:
Leg extension

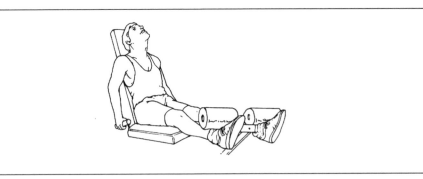

Leg Curls

Lie on the floor, with your arms at your side and the weights around your ankles. Turn your head to one side and lift both feet toward your buttocks, bringing your heels as close to your buttocks as you can (see

FIGURE 8-11). Use your abs to keep your hips pressing into the floor and lower your legs to the starting position for one rep.

FIGURE 8-11:
Leg curl

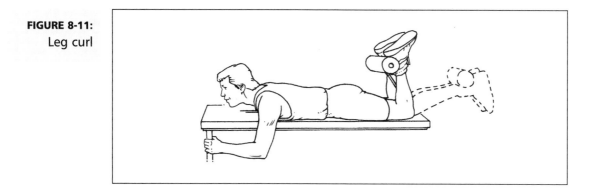

Abs and Back

Use the following exercises to strengthen your abdominal and back muscles. You could do some of these every day, so long as you don't overdo it.

Pelvic Tilt

Laying on your back on the floor, preferably on a mat or folded towel for some cushion, bend your knees, rest your heels on the floor, and let your toes point up. Keep your arms at your side. Imagine gravity pulling your bellybutton into the floor so that your lower back is flattened against the floor. This will cause your pelvis to raise slightly and you should feel your abs tighten (see **FIGURE 8-12**). Hold this position for several seconds, then relax and repeat. Do three sets of ten reps.

FIGURE 8-12:
Posterior
pelvic tilt

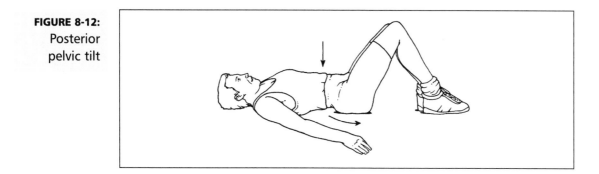

Abdominal Crunch

You've probably seen the technique for doing crunches explained several ways. Forget the others and follow this one. Lie on your back with your knees bent and feet flat on the floor, about shoulder-width apart. Bring your arms up and put your hands under your head, thumbs pointing toward your ears. Don't interlock your fingers, even if your fingers overlap. Keep your head extended from your body so that your chin isn't digging into your chest. Start raising your trunk, curling up from your spine, using your abs—not your hands—to pull you up.

Keep your elbows to the side and raise yourself up only enough to lift your shoulder blades off the floor (see **FIGURE 8-13**). Pause, then bring your trunk back into position slowly for one repetition. Start by doing three sets of fifteen reps, adjusting according to whether it feels like too much or not enough.

To increase the intensity of your ab crunch workout, try doing your reps with your legs off the floor, crossed at your ankles. Keep your knees bent and your butt on the floor.

FIGURE 8-13:
Abdominal
crunch

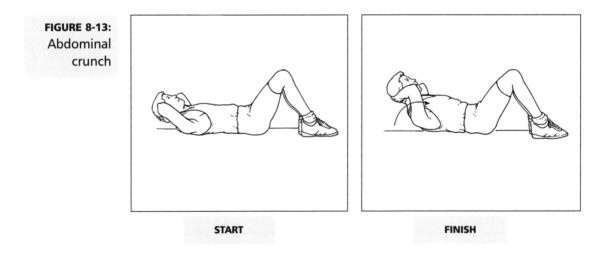

START   FINISH

ESSENTIALS Rather than lifting heavy weights only a few times like body builders and power lifters do, emphasize lighter weights and more repetitions (twelve to fifteen). Don't overdo exercises that will leave your legs fatigued for your next run. Instead, concentrate your efforts on your upper body and carefully chose the lower extremity exercises that work for you.

Remember These Weight Training Tips

To have a successful weight training experience, keep the following guidelines in mind:

- Warm up before lifting and stretch thoroughly afterward.
- Run prior to lifting and avoid weight training leg work on days before races, speed workouts, or long runs.
- Lift every other day or a minimum of three days per week.
- Emphasize lighter weights and more repetitions rather than heavy weights a few reps.
- Don't hold your breath while lifting weights; breathe in on the relaxation phase and out while performing the hard part of the exercise.
- Move your body through the entire range of motion of the exercise, making sure you don't "lock" your joints while performing the exercise.
- Follow the sequence of legs first, upper body second, and midsection last, remembering to work your abdominal muscles.
- In each sequence, exercise the larger muscle groups first, followed by the smaller groups.

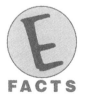

FACTS Remember, you probably won't lose weight as you infuse a weight-conditioning program into your present training. Instead, you will lose body fat (assuming you eat sensibly); thus the scales can be very misleading. As you lose fat and gain muscle, your clothes will fit better, and you'll look and feel great!

Run First, Lift Later

Runners should ideally run first and do strength training second, preferably not back to back. The best thing to do is schedule several hours between the run and your strength workout. You may run in the morning and then do your strength routine at lunchtime or in the evening. If you are forced to perform the two routines together, do your run first and then your strength training. If you're doing a long run or speed workout, hold off on the strength training afterward. You'll probably be too tired to perform it properly.

Some have recommended that you can perform your hard running and strength training on the same day (but separate the two), followed by an easy run the next day since you'll have time to recover. Experiment to see what feels right to you. You might find that it is easier to do your strength training on a light running day or a cross-training day or even on a "rest" day. For more advanced runners, if you do strength training on a rest day, go very easy on the legs or skip legs entirely if you will be racing or doing a speed work session the next day.

Cross-Training

Over the past few years, runners of all abilities have discovered the many benefits of cross-training as a means to enhance total conditioning and running performance. Yet despite cross-training's recent popularity, some runners still wonder why they should participate in aerobic activities other than running.

Although cross-training can provide numerous benefits, too much of a good thing can be counterproductive and detrimental to one's running. For example, partaking in certain cross-training activities on a scheduled rest day may leave one tired prior to attempting an important workout, such as a long run (especially for those in training for races such as a half-marathon or marathon).

Furthermore, some cross-training activities can actually increase the likelihood of an injury, particularly during the mileage buildup stage. This in turn may prevent a runner from completing the training necessary to obtain his/her running goals of participating in and finishing events of any distance from the 5K to the marathon. After reading this section, pick and choose your cross-training activities carefully and schedule these sessions to enhance, rather than detract from, your running goals.

Benefits and Purposes of Cross-Training

One of the great benefits of cross-training is that it adds variety to your training and decreases the chance of burnout. Cross-training can occasionally be substituted for "easy day" running (as an aerobic workout). Cross-training can serve as an injury prevention measure. In fact, certain activities such as cycling can strengthen related muscle groups and soft connective tissue.

Of course, one of the great benefits of cross-training is that it provides an extra way to burn fat. Many cross-training activities such as rowing or using the VersaClimber help increase upper body strength. Upper body strength is very important in races of all distances as neck and shoulder muscles often become fatigued. Upper body strength is also important in ascending hills.

Precautions and Considerations

Remember, cross-training is not intended to replace running but rather to enhance and supplement it. For example, a ninety-minute run shouldn't be substituted with a ninety-minute bike ride. This is the concept of sports specificity. A ninety-minute bike ride won't provide the training effect needed to run a longer race such as a half-marathon.

ALERT

Use common sense when deciding whether to add certain sports to your fitness regimen. Avoid high-impact fitness routines, especially those with quick or sudden movements. Don't participate strenuously in the following sports, as doing so can traumatize the soft connective tissue that surrounds the knees and ankles: tennis, racquetball, basketball, soccer, volleyball, downhill skiing, kick-boxing, and aerobic dance.

Rest Days

Designate at least one day a week, preferably two, as complete leg rest days. This is particularly important prior to long runs, races, and fast-paced training runs when it's crucial to be as rested as possible.

Great Cross-Training Activities

The following are cross-training activities that are ideally suited to enhance your running performance. They are recommended because they are all north-south exercises, which place little side-to-side lateral pressures on your body, especially your leg joints, muscles, and connective tissue. While these cross-training activities offer great cardiovascular workouts, they also give the legs a heavy-duty workout and thus should not be done on scheduled leg rest days.

Cycling

Cycling exercises some of the same muscle groups as running, such as the quadriceps and shins, both of which don't develop as rapidly as the calf muscles and hamstrings. Cycling also strengthens the connective tissue of the knee, hip, and ankle regions, thus reducing the risk of injury. After a stressful run, cycling can loosen fatigued leg muscles.

There are three types of biking to try: road riding, mountain biking, or stationary cycling. Road biking takes place on the road and allows you to travel long distances with speed. Mountain bikes are two-wheel, all-terrain vehicles that can be ridden almost anywhere. While mountain biking is a lot of fun and challenging, road and/or stationary cycling are much better alternatives; mountain biking is much more risky due the possibility of falls and its jarring nature. With stationary cycling, you can work out indoors year-round, regardless of inclement weather conditions. Extra benefits of stationary cycling are also that you can safely listen to music or read when doing this.

A few things to remember: If at all possible, refrain from cycling on a scheduled rest day. Since it's much more difficult to run after cycling, run prior to heading out on your bike. Spin easily, as opposed to grinding big gears. Be sure that your seat height and pedals are properly positioned. Finally, always wear a helmet and leave the Walkman at home!

ESSENTIALS

Remember these cycling tips: First, always maintain control of your bike. To slow down or stop, "feather" the brakes, alternating between squeezing and releasing them. Also, be aware of cars. Don't assume drivers see you. When you ride past parked cars, watch for car doors opening suddenly. Additionally, know bicycling etiquette. Observe traffic signals/signs and use hand signals to indicate turns or stops.

Water Activities

For the compulsive athlete, swimming is one of the best cross-training activities to add to his or her regimen. Swimming enables a runner to give tired leg muscles a breather while providing an excellent upper body workout. Additionally, water provides a therapeutic effect for all muscle groups. Although gentle kicking alleviates some muscle soreness and fatigue, avoid using the kickboard for hard kick sets on your running rest day.

If you swim for the aerobic benefit, do not be concerned that your heart rate does not get as high as it does during other activities. The loss of gravitational force, the horizontal position, and the cooling effect of the water temperature all contribute toward keeping your heart rate low.

A low heart rate does not mean that your aerobic efforts are in vain. Remember, aerobic exercise is about oxygen utilization, and the heart rate is just a mirror for what is happening on an oxygen level. But in this case, the mirror is reflecting a hazy and distorted picture of what's really going on. Even though the conditions in swimming produce relatively lower heart rate numbers, your body is still processing oxygen, and that's what counts. A general rule is that the swimming heart rate is typically ten to twenty beats per minute less than what it is for dry land activities.

Another type of water cross-training activity is deep water running. In deep water running, you are suspended in a pool vertically through the use of a flotation belt worn around your waist or torso. With your feet not touching the bottom of the pool, you then simulate running.

This cross-training activity is just what the doctor ordered for the rehabilitation of many running injuries. Because there is no shock from footstrike, water running is a great alternative to a midweek "easy day" run. The idea is that you get all the benefits of running with the resistance of the water and none of the shock and pounding of footstrike associated with road running. While it is possible to run in the water without floatation aids, find a pool that has these devices (for instance, vests, belts, etc.) to make your workout both easier on your upper body and more specific in targeting your leg muscles.

Exercise Machines

One popular cross-training machine is the egrometer, or rowing machine. As scullers have known for centuries, rowing is a terrific all-body exercise, utilizing strength from your back, buttocks, and legs and driving power from your shoulders and arms. Now people who've never been in a shell on the water can reap the same benefits and can do so indoors to boot!

Rowing involves a two-stroke movement—the drive and the recovery, which are blended together to create a smooth and continuous action. It's important to follow good form on a rowing machine, so make sure you ask your health club to show you how to use it properly. This is another great activity that can be done on a rest day. It strengthens the hips, buttocks, and upper body while sparing the legs of heavy pounding.

In addition to rowing machines, you can also try the Nordic Track and other ski-simulator machines. Designed to simulate cross-country skiing, these machines, when used properly, are highly effective in building aerobic conditioning, muscular strength, and endurance. In short, they provide an excellent workout for runners. The dual action movement of the upper and lower body challenges your ability to balance and coordinate two different movements.

The Stair Master, stair stepper, or "stepper" can be thought of as the next generation of running the bleachers or the stairwells. It's a machine that simulates climbing stairs, and you can adjust it to the level of workout you want to put in. In addition to getting the average person fit, these stair-climbing simulators provide a terrific cross-training exercise that will more than sufficiently augment running or walking. Climbing stairs is gentle upon the skeletal system, and many love this activity for its ability to challenge them aerobically while giving their bones and joints a rest.

More complex than the stair stepper, the VersaClimber is the ultimate fat burner because it can work all the major muscles of the upper and lower body, all while climbing against gravity. It is one of the most difficult machines to use in the gym, but once you've mastered it, you will invest less time while burning more calories then on bikes, steppers, treadmills, or ski machines.

A VersaClimber can be used in two ways. You can have a lower body workout, where you use the handrails and use the step portion only. Or, you can grab hold of the handles that are attached about chest high and that reach well above the head and begin "climbing" as you would on a ladder. It is this workout that provides a total body workout. And like most of the cross-training workouts mentioned here, it is a straightforward workout that is excellent for runners.

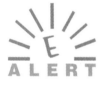

Proper stair climbing posture is when the back is erect, arms are bent yet relaxed, hands and wrists are in an overhand position and used only to balance, feet are fully on the pads, and the legs extend down to an almost straight stance. Avoid leaning over the machine, which can cause backache, lower leg soreness, and wrist and shoulder injury.

Walking

That's right, good old walking is a great way to cross-train. It's an underrated activity that provides great therapeutic benefits following a long run or speed work. While walking is not a substitute for an easy running day, a relaxed two- to three-mile stroll is a great way to loosen up the legs the day prior to a big race. Depending on the type of injury, speed-walking is a great rehabilitation activity to maintain cardiovascular fitness.

CHAPTER 9

On the Road All Year

As you've probably realized by now, running is something you can do any time of the year. But running intelligently during the different seasons requires forethought and specific strategies, especially during the extreme seasons of winter and summer. This chapter will take you through the practical and medical information necessary to deal with the elements and enjoy your sport all year round.

Running in Cold Weather

Depending upon your geographic location, winter may not be the optimal time to plan a dramatic increase in mileage or to add speed work to your training regimen. Cold and icy conditions make running more hazardous. Slipping, muscle guarding, and cool muscles may contribute to posterior muscle group and groin pulls.

Cold Weather Strategies

Warm up well before going out and be especially careful when running on surfaces that are wet or icy. Shorten your stride and run slower than usual. When running just after a winter storm, if you have a choice of running on ice or snow, choose the snow. You will be less likely to slip because the traction is better.

To help yourself keep warm, a good strategy to remember is to run out against the wind and return with the wind at your back. The greater the amount of cold air passing over your exposed body surface, the faster your body will cool off. By running against the wind, you'll be facing the greatest environmental cooling stresses when you are fresh and running faster. When you are fatigued at the end of a run and expending less energy, you will be producing less body heat and thereby have a greater tendency for your core temperature to drop. The wind behind you will help keep you moving.

Dressing for Cold Weather Runs

It is important to protect all areas of your body from exposure. This includes your head, hands, feet, legs, arms, and chest. Also, don't forget your private parts. Men may want to consider investing in underwear with an insulated front panel for extra protection.

To protect your feet, which conduct cold through the soles of your running shoes as they strike the cold trails or roads, wear absorbent and dry socks. In many cases, polypropylene or acrylic can wick moisture away, which will prevent moisture from forming around your feet while you run and turning to ice when you stop running. A thin inner sock can be covered with a thicker outer sock, provided it doesn't pad your foot so much that you can barely squeeze your foot into your shoe. Immediately following your run, change into a dry pair of socks.

Polypropylene and Gore-tex are highly effective materials that offer protection for keeping your body warm and dry. Combined with a lightweight Gore-tex suit, you can run comfortably without having to wear multiple layers of T-shirts, sweatshirts, and parkas. When it isn't too cold, a single layer of a polypropylene shirt below a sweatshirt should be enough for your upper body, and polypropylene or lycra tights should suffice for your legs.

When it becomes very cold, Gore-tex or nylon will help lessen the effect of wind chill. Use an inner layer of polypropylene and, optionally, a long-sleeved T-shirt as a middle layer, then as the outer layer, a Gore-tex or nylon windbreaker. For the legs, you may add sweat pants over polypropylene tights or, if it is exceptionally cold, wear Gore-tex or nylon pants for the outer layer.

On very cold days, no matter how long you plan to run and especially for longer workouts, don't forget to cover your head and your hands. For your head, choose a lightweight synthetic fabric that will wick away moisture and won't itch. For your hands, some runners use the Bill Rodgers–recommended painters gloves for relatively mild temperatures. For colder weather, inner polypropylene gloves and an outer layer of mittens can be worn.

ESSENTIALS
Your skin is the part of your body that is most exposed to the environmental conditions in which you run. Nourish and protect it by staying hydrated whether it's hot or cold out and wear a sunscreen when you run. Sun block and moisturizer will help prevent the development of a grizzled, weather-worn-looking face.

Running in Hot Weather

The best defense against heat is hydration. Therefore when the temperature goes up, so should your fluid intake. Water should always be your number-one drink of choice. Drink before, during, and after you run.

Drink before you go to sleep, and drink when you wake up. In short, drink water often throughout the day, regardless of weather conditions. In general, you should drink at least eight glasses of water a day. When it's really hot out, you could easily double this amount.

Always drink before you run and try to drink about eight ounces every twenty-five minutes while you run. Water is just fine for runs of up to an hour, but you will find that sports drinks maintain your performance level for runs over one hour. Most popular sport drinks have a low level of electrolytes and also contain carbohydrates (both simple and more complex polymers) to help speed up glycogen replacement.

Please don't count coffee, beer, or other caffeinated or alcoholic beverages among your daily tally of fluids. Caffeine and alcohol act as diuretics and will cause an overall fluid loss.

ALERT

According to research studies, caffeine does seem to enhance performance. You may not want to skip it before you run, but make sure you drink plenty of water, too. Coffee is a diuretic and a dehydrator. And depending on how long your run is, remember that the caffeine "buzz" can turn into a drop.

Immediately following exercise, the muscles are most receptive to absorbing carbohydrates sources (which later converts to glycogen in the muscles), which is why you'll often find bagels and PowerBars or other sports bars offered at the end of a race. But don't forget your overall fluid replacement needs should be met with water as well as fluids containing ample carbohydrates, such as fruit or vegetable juices.

To help you stay hydrated during long, hot summers of running, you might consider stopping at every water fountain you pass and taking a drink. Don't forget to give yourself a minimum of two weeks to acclimate to the heat. The best way to do this is by running a slow three to four miles, making sure you've had enough water. Increase your distance and cumulative time running gradually.

Also try combining treadmill running and outside running to get more distance on the really hot days. During those first hot, humid days of spring and summer, slowly build your mileage to acclimate to these conditions before considering running at a faster pace. In fact, many seasoned runners put their fast-paced efforts on hold until the cooler weather returns. Additionally, try to just plain miss the heat by running early in the morning or late at night. Remember though that if you run early in the morning, you may experience more humidity. And of course you can consider using a treadmill on the worst days. This way you can get a workout and a few more miles in a cooler environment.

FACTS

Perspiration and evaporation of perspiration are the primary means for the body to cool during exercise. Sweat glands become active as body core temperature rises. One liter of sweat is generated during the expenditure of about 500 kcal. Skin blood flow also increases significantly during exercise. Blood flowing near the surface results in cooling by both conduction and convection.

Heat-Induced Illness

Several different kinds of illnesses can be induced by heat. The first, heat exhaustion, is caused by dehydration. The symptoms include chills, lightheadedness, dizziness, headache, and nausea. The body temperature is usually between 100–102 degrees Fahrenheit and profuse sweating is evident. To treat heat exhaustion, move the individual to a cool, shaded area and administer fluids either by mouth, if conscious, or by IV if the individual is unconscious. Then, seek medical advice.

Heat stroke, another type of heat-induced illness, is caused by a sudden failure of the body's thermoregulatory system. Not only is this dangerous, but it can also be fatal. Heat stroke initially displays similar to heat exhaustion but may rapidly progress to more serious neurological symptoms, such as disorientation, loss of consciousness, and seizures. The body temperature may be higher than 104 degrees Fahrenheit. Sweating is often absent, but the skin may be quite moist from earlier perspiration. The pulse of the afflicted person is usually over 160 beats per minute, and blood pressure may be low.

Someone suffering from heat stroke must have his or her core temperature reduced immediately. Kidney damage (acute nephropathy) occurs in about 35 percent of cases. This is a result of *rhabdomyolysis* (muscle breakdown) and the *myoglobulinuria* (excretion of muscle breakdown products), which contributes to the kidney injury. Liver damage is also evident when liver enzymes are measured following heatstroke. Oftentimes, core temperature is reduced by the individual getting packed in ice. If heat stroke is suspected, rapid medical attention is vital.

Avoiding Heat Stress Injury

To avoid heat exhaustion or heat stroke, drink plenty of fluids (preferably water) twenty-five to thirty minutes before exercise and then eight ounces every twenty-five to thirty minutes while exercising. After exercising, drink more fluids than you think you need, especially if you are over the age of forty. Don't wait until you feel thirsty; by that time you're dehydrated. Drinking fluid while you exercise as well as when you're finished will help speed your recovery.

You can also protect yourself from the heat by gradually building up your tolerance for running in warmer weather. Stay fit and don't overestimate your level of fitness. Individuals with a higher VO_2 max (how much oxygen your body can transport to your muscles every minute) are more tolerant of heat than those with a lower level of fitness.

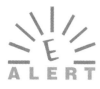

Make sure you are aware of any medical conditions or medications you are taking that can affect your tolerance for exercise in the heat. Medical conditions affecting heat tolerance include diabetes, high blood pressure, anorexia nervosa, bulimia, obesity, and fever.

Dressing Cool for the Heat

You're going to feel like you don't want to wear anything at all when it's really hot out but don't make that mistake! The worst thing to do is overheat your body and then, with no protection, expose it to rapid cooling. This can cause faint-headedness and dizziness.

When running in the heat, wear lightweight fabrics that wick away moisture. There are all sorts of comfortable and fashionable shorts available for men and women. As for upper body wear, women can opt for a colorful sports bra and men a breezy fabric singlet. Thin, absorbent socks will keep your feet from getting too sweaty, and to keep the sweat from pouring into your eyes, you may want to wear a headband or a visor. While baseball caps do shield the sun, they trap heat—something to consider on those hot humid days. Don't forget to apply heavy-duty sunscreen, especially on your face.

Play It Safe

The message of this chapter is to warn you that running in extreme temperatures can be dangerous. That said, if you use common sense, dress correctly, stay hydrated, and follow the normal protocol of letting someone know your running route and not overexerting yourself on your training runs, you should be able to stick to a training schedule through all seasons. There's no excuse for not being prepared and learning about what tomorrow's weather is going to be like when you run.

ESSENTIALS

It is important to remember that environmental comfort is a highly individualized matter. By experimenting with a variety of apparel and layering options, you will learn how to dress effectively and comfortably in facing the elements. This in turn will enable you to train both safely and consistently.

Running Indoors

As mentioned before, running outside in inclement weather is a good thing because it prepares you for races, which don't stop for the weather (save of course for extreme weather, like hurricanes, snow storms, etc.). Running outside regardless of the weather is a healthy and invigorating experience.

Even so, realize also that running indoors is reliable, convenient, limits your exposure to outside risks, and can be more social if you choose it to be. Running indoors can be done at home, or at a gym or club, usually using a treadmill. There are new indoor treadmills coming to market all the time. The best indoor treadmill is the one that works for you. Experiment with several before you hone in on one or two and be receptive to trying the new ones that show up in your gym.

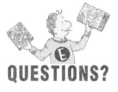

QUESTIONS?

How do I know my miles per hour?
Pace is the number of minutes it takes to travel one mile. To determine your pace, divide 60 by your speed in miles per hour. For example: If your treadmill speed equals 3.5 mph, divide 60 by 3.5. You are running a 17-minute mile!

Running on treadmills is recommended when you have no choice and you don't want to miss a workout. The treadmill's convenience is wonderful, but it will not help you train for long-distance running in the end. Those in training for a marathon still have to do a large percentage of running on the roads, particularly for those all-important long runs. As you run indoors, remember to continue focusing on your form. When you exercise, proper posture and technique are essential to maximizing your effort and avoiding injury. Many runners respect the importance of posture and mechanics when doing outside sports but give little thought to it when exercising indoors on equipment. Consider this; it matters.

Using the Treadmill

Most commercial equipment in health clubs is clearly labeled with instructions. But if you are still unclear about how to use the equipment, ask the staff for assistance. If you are going to buy a piece of equipment, make sure you get a demonstration (and a warranty and instruction manual if buying from a retail store) on how to properly use and maintain it.

Here are some tips for using a treadmill:

1. Learn how to use it *before* you use it.
2. Use manual mode for complete control of the intensity (speed, elevation, and resistances).
3. Pay attention to your intensity level and using distractions (music, reading, talking, thinking) to pass the time so you don't overdo it.
4. Drink water during exercise to stay hydrated.
5. Use a fan to keep from getting overheated.

Once you get used to the feeling of the ground moving beneath your feet, you can truly appreciate running on a treadmill. The treadmill is obedient and will keep the speed and elevation steady at the levels you set. Intensity is determined by the speed and elevation settings. You can either control the settings yourself through the manual mode or experiment with the preprogrammed workouts. Many home models will allow you to program your own workouts and keep them in memory as a preprogrammed workout.

ESSENTIALS

Learn how to control your treadmill:

- Know where the stop button is located.
- Practice grabbing the handrail and standing on the nonmoving side panels before stopping the machine.
- Stay focused and avoid turning your body or looking directly down at your feet.
- Keep children and pets away from the treadmill and from the operating key.
- Position the back of the treadmill away from a wall so that you do not bump into it.

Shopping for a Treadmill

Commercial treadmills can accommodate persons of most body weights; home models are typically built to withstand body weights not greater than 250 pounds. If you presently walk and are planning to eventually run on the treadmill, a minimum horsepower of 1.5 to 2.0 is recommended. Be sure to ask the salesperson if the machine has elevation change capability. Elevation capability gives you more variety in the types of workouts you can do or progress into doing.

Noise is difficult to detect on the showroom floor but listen for it anyway. Compare the surroundings to those where you may put your machine. If it seems a bit noisy in the showroom and you plan to put the treadmill in a small room with little insulation, expect that it will be even louder at home.

Take measurements to make sure you have enough room for the treadmill you are considering, and for safety purposes, avoid positioning the treadmill with its back close to a wall. One small misstep and you could be thrown into an unplanned back injury, as well as finding yourself in need of some home remodeling.

Safety Features

You absolutely want an emergency pull/stop mechanism. In the event that you would unexpectedly fall (or move more than a few feet from the treadmill), a light emergency cord connected to the treadmill control panel would disengage and instantly stop the motor. Some people prefer to wear it clipped onto their clothing; others prefer for it to rest within reach on top of the treadmill. Either is an effective and valuable safety feature.

Another safety factor and personal preference for many people is the treadmill railing. Front rails are best; side rails are steadying but, for some, can get in the way during exercise. If you aren't sure which you prefer, this is another reason to check out several treadmills and feel the differences between the models.

Deck, Speed, and Other Features

Deck flexibility will make a difference in how your bones and joints feel in response to the impact. There is no standard word to describe how flexible the deck is, but you need to inquire if the treadmills you are considering have such a system. Good treadmills have some type of flexible deck system.

You also want a smooth belt action, which means that the machine can pull its own weight (and yours) without hesitation or knocking. Ask what the maximum speed and maximum elevation of the machine are. If you consistently run a blazing six-minute mile or faster, some treadmills cannot match your speed, and therefore, you would not want to buy them.

The components panel may display your distance, speed, calories burned, elevation, programmable workouts, and heart rate monitor. The more components you want to see displayed on the console, the higher the price. But do not let that discourage you. Envision yourself walking and running on the treadmill for years to come and think about how much enjoyment and motivation you will derive from knowing how you performed in those seemingly trivial areas that the console displays.

Lastly, note which creature comforts, if any, are important to you, such as cup and magazine holders. Make a list of questions and bring it with you when shopping so that all of your concerns are addressed before buying.

Do not waste your money on non-electrical or human-powered treadmills. They have a limited capacity for generating any degree of exercise happiness and satisfaction. The movement of the belt is stiff, sluggish, and uneven and it doesn't feel like something you'd want to stay on for more than one minute. The mental and physical energy spent on it can be better spent on something more enjoyable and easier to use.

CHAPTER 10
On the Road to Speed

How can I increase my speed? Most runners ask this question once they become more accomplished. Indeed, one of the best things about running is being able to compete not only against others but also against yourself. Improvement is almost always possible, but it is also always illusory. If you run faster this week, can you run even faster next? Runners have been asking this question since the Greeks staged the first Olympics, and probably before.

Adding Speed Work to Your Running Program

Incorporating some carefully designed faster-paced runs is an essential component of a program that will yield faster performances in your daily training runs or in races you wish to enter. However, the key point to remember is that speed work is an advanced training technique for the experienced runner and not for the true beginner.

For the more accomplished runner, though, incorporating some advanced running techniques is essential if you want to improve your time from one race to the next. One's best race times are referred to as PRs (personal records) or PBs (personal bests).

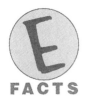

FACTS

PR (personal record) and PB (personal best) both represent a runner's fastest time posted at a given distance. For a runner to claim a PR or PB, the run must be done on a track or a road race course that has been certified as accurate by the USA Track and Field (USATF), the national governing body for track and field, long-distance running, and race walking.

In short, don't entertain the notion of adding speed work to your training regimen until you have been running regularly (logging twenty to twenty-five miles per week) for a minimum of a year. Doing so without this solid mileage base greatly increases your chances of incurring an injury. If you do decide to focus on this aspect of your running, it is important to read this entire section before beginning any speed workouts on your own.

The Risks

Despite the benefit of increasing your speed, infusing advanced training techniques exponentially increases your risk of injury. You really need to think about whether you are willing (after weeks and/or months of training) to risk injury that may prevent you from participating in your chosen event.

Runners who feel they are ready to work on and improve their speed still need to be careful. Speed workouts are sessions where, yes, you need to push yourself. But pushing too hard may result in injury. You have to be smart. Exert yourself, as there is no gain without some physical discomfort, but don't be macho. A mistake here can result in serious, if not languorous, injuries that may keep you from running for weeks and even months at a time.

The Benefits

There are many benefits from adding advanced running techniques to your training, well beyond merely improving your speed and chocking up faster race times. These benefits are both physical and mental.

Physical Gains

The physical gains obtained through speed work are more numerous than you might think. There's the obvious, which of course is improved strength and speed. However, that's actually a byproduct of the training. With higher intensity training, you now have a better oxygen delivery system. You can run faster and still stay at a comfortable, aerobic (meaning using air) pace. Your body will become more efficient at delivering oxygen to your muscles, and your muscles will function better while utilizing less oxygen.

When your body exceeds its capacity to use oxygen as its fuel, you will begin using glycogen as your primary fuel source. A byproduct of this anaerobic (without oxygen) method of energy production is lactic acid. Rather than your body going into "oxygen debt" (characterized by that heavy, burning feeling in your legs), where your muscles tie up due to a buildup of lactic acid from a lack of oxygen, your anaerobic system can be trained like your cardiovascular system was trained. With specific anaerobic training, you can exceed limits that previously held you back.

Fine-Tuning Your Mechanics

If you train diligently, your running mechanics will surely improve, especially if you've been able to work with and implement the recommendations of a running coach or experienced runners. Your arm drive, your stride, and your breathing will all improve as a result of incorporating advanced running techniques into your training. You will run faster with less effort during your daily runs, and your speed will improve for races you wish to enter.

A competent coach can usually be found through running clubs, a specialty running store, college or university, or on the Web. Before you commit to a particular coach, ask lots of questions about the coach's background and training philosophy. Be sure that the one you choose will be the right one for you.

Mental Edge

The mental benefits of doing speed work are much like the benefits for doing any kind of running with the added benefit of setting and achieving time-related goals. Running PRs off your improved speed are quite fulfilling and can be highly motivating. Speed work can be challenging and sometimes quite uncomfortable; perhaps even painful (not to be confused with the pain associated with injury, however).

You are asking your body to perform faster and outside of the aerobic zone, which through training has become comfortable on long, slow runs. You're pushing the limits of your body and mind, pushing past old physical and mental barriers. The end result is that your mental toughness will improve significantly, both during fast-paced training runs and when competing in races of all distances.

Race Strategy

Last, but certainly not least, is the benefit of planning and implementing a smart race day strategy. Your speed workouts will furnish you with improved stamina throughout the entire race, which alone will result in a better finish time. A smart race strategy means planning your race in advance. Rather than sprinting through the first part of a 5K as if you're competing in the Olympic 100 meter finals and having little energy left for the rest of the race, your experience from running intervals on the track will give you a good idea of what pace you can and should run during a race.

Quick Guidelines for Speed Work

Please refer to other sections of this and other chapters within this book for a comprehensive discussion on general training principles, stretching, and injury prevention strategies, among other topics that also relate to advanced running techniques. Some basic guidelines for speed work are as follows.

First, you should be consistently running a minimum of twenty to twenty-five miles per week for a year before you even begin to think about including advanced training techniques to your training schedule. If you've never included speed work as part of your training, learn as much as you can from credible sources (books, magazine articles, Web sites, etc.) so that you have the knowledge you need to train smart. It is important to confirm that this information is accurate and up to date and from reliable sources.

Be sure to follow the *hard-easy concept of training* if you intend to integrate speed training into your program. For example, do not schedule a speed work session the day after a long run or after participating in a road race. Assuming that their longest run of the week is Sunday, most experienced runners do their speed training during the middle days of the week following an easy run or a complete leg rest day.

If you choose to participate in speed work with a group, be sure to run at a pace that is appropriate for your ability level. Trying to perform a workout designed for someone else (in particular, runners who are significantly faster than you are) greatly increases your chances of incurring an injury and can also be discouraging. To avoid injury, proper warm-ups and cool-downs are essential. These include light jogging and stretching both before and after the workout.

No more than 15 to 20 percent of your total weekly mileage should be fast-paced running. This percentage reflects both speed workouts as well as races. The volume of your fast-paced running should not be increased by more than 800 meters per week.

If you elect to do speed workouts during the summer months, schedule them for the early morning or evening to avoid the most hot/humid times of the day. Pushing the pace in these conditions increases your chances succumbing to various degrees of heat illness.

Finally, be careful of what you eat and how soon you time your meals and snacks before fast-paced running. Experimenting with a variety of foods and drinks is the best way to determine what your system can tolerate. Don't eat a big lunch if you're planning on doing a fast-paced run later in the afternoon. Instead, have small snacks throughout the day.

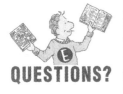

QUESTIONS?

What are the benefits of doing speed work with a group?
"Doing speed work in a group helps you push yourself. It gives you a sense of competition. It also gives people more inspiration. People feel better in groups. They are more apt to push themselves as they see other people pushing themselves. Misery loves company."

—Pam Spadola, Howell, NJ, speed work group leader, Freehold Area Running Club

Overview of Advanced Training

Speed work can be uncomfortable and, yes, sometimes even painful. Often, while listening to the objections coming from your lungs and legs, there's a little voice inside your head saying, "What is this all about? Let's stop this pain right now and have ourselves a fudge sundae." But the fact of the matter is that by doing speed workouts, you will be able to quiet that voice by becoming accustomed to running faster and tolerating both the physical and mental discomforts when racing. In quieting that voice, you will also be able to run faster during your easy training runs without any extra effort due to your improved cardiovascular conditioning.

Through speed work, you can improve your body's ability to run faster with limited oxygen stores available. Additionally, your speed will improve on your easier runs. Like anything else, you need to apply stress in small progressive steps over a period of weeks. Just like weightlifters will work up to a new weight slowly (they don't just walk into the gym and haphazardly slap twenty-five to thirty extra pounds on the bar) or swimmers increase their ability to hold their breath, runners' bodies must gradually adapt to the stress of running fast to improve their tolerance to lactic acid buildup. This is the purpose of speed work.

The Physiological Aspects of Speed Training

Everyone knows that when you sprint or climb a few flights of stairs you get a burning sensation in your legs. This feeling occurs due to your muscles working while being deprived of oxygen. During everyday activities and long, slow running, your body uses mostly oxygen as fuel (aerobic running). As you increase the workload on your muscles, your body will begin burning stored fuel, called glycogen, for energy. This anaerobic (without oxygen) workout results in an accumulation of lactic acid, which is a byproduct of anaerobic metabolism. With continued effortful movement, this lactic acid will accumulate to the point where it will begin shutting down your muscles.

The point at which your body reaches its maximum capacity for utilizing oxygen and then switches over to accumulating lactic acid is termed the anaerobic threshold. With proper speed training this threshold can be raised, which allows you to run at a faster pace before reaching the point where lactic acid accumulation begins slowing you down.

Another important factor that relates to running performance is your aerobic capacity. This value, also known as your max VO_2, or maximal oxygen uptake, is a measure of how well your body utilizes large volumes of oxygen during your peak performances. An apparatus used in human performance labs measures your max VO_2 while you run all out on a treadmill.

There are some other inherited qualities that can either work for or against you. Your morphology (body type), the ratio of your fast twitch to slow twitch muscle fibers (those who excel at sprinting have higher ratios of fast twitch muscle fibers as opposed to those who perform better in endurance events, who have a higher ratio of slow twitch muscle fibers), and the quality of your cardio-respiratory system all play roles in how well you are able to reach your full potential as a runner. Like your aerobic capacity and anaerobic threshold, most genetic attributes can be minimized or enhanced through proper training.

ESSENTIALS

One of the best ways to do speed work with others is to contact a local running club. One way to find a running club is to contact the Road Runners Club of America (*www.rrca.org*) for a list of running clubs throughout the nation. Many running clubs hold weekly speed workout sessions at a local track and sometimes offer seminars at club meetings.

When Do I Begin My Speed Work?

If you want to pull it all together and train seriously for a race, don't start too early or too late. You should only train intensely for three to four months at a time. Additionally, one can usually only peak (race your best) two or three times a year. Overdoing it with speed work week after week can lead to excessive fatigue and burnout. To establish a baseline to determine your present race pace, enter a 5K or 10K race. Then begin your "prime-time training" three to four months prior to the race at which you want to achieve your best performance.

Where Do I Run My Speed Workout?

The best possible place to do speed work is at a local outdoor track. These can be found at a local park, high school, or college. It is worth your while to travel the distance to one of these facilities to do your speed work.

Why do you need to use a real track? You should seek out an existing track because the heart of speed workouts are comprised of short segments of distances from 200 to 1,600 meters. Tracks are accurately measured so you know exactly how far you are running as well as your exact pace.

Although it's not essential, the best track to use is one with a synthetic or rubberized surface. Unlike a cinder or asphalt track, the softer surface of a synthetic track is preferable because it's easier on your legs. Oftentimes the surface of a dirt or cinder track is not consistently smooth, which increases the risk of foot and ankle injuries. Running speed work on dirt and cinder surfaces will also add a few seconds to your lap times.

A quick word about indoor tracks: One must run several more laps to the mile indoors compared to four times around an outdoor track. The turns on indoor tracks are also much tighter than outdoor tracks, which can wreak havoc on your knees if you aren't used to them. However, in the winter, an indoor track can be a safe, dry haven for dodging the elements.

If you can't get to a track, find a safe place to lay out a running loop for yourself. Try using a bicycle with a cyclo-computer rather than a car odometer to measure your route. There are also new pedometer-like products on the market now (Nike and FitSense are two manufacturers) that measure both one's pace and distance covered. A sensor chip attached to the running shoe relays highly accurate pace-distance information to an accompanying watch.

Because you will be running short distance segments such as 200, 400, and 800 meters, you want the mileage marked out to be as accurate as possible. Mileage estimated from a car odometer would be inaccurate, making your times less meaningful. You will be expending both physical effort and mental energy when doing speed work. Therefore, try to find a place where there won't be lots of obstacles or distractions such as streets with heavy traffic or paths with lots of bikes and pedestrians—things that can steal some of the mental focus needed for high-intensity workouts.

ALERT

For all beginners and novice runners, you should not run more than one speed work session a week. The idea of speed work is that over time you gradually stress your anaerobic and cardio-vascular systems in progressive increments.

CHAPTER 11

Advanced Running Workouts

There are a wide variety of workouts that encompass advanced training techniques. The most common workouts include hill repeats, fartlek runs, striders (also called pickups), tempo runs, and even road races. When integrated carefully into one's training (based on ability level and goals), these workouts can make you a stronger and faster runner.

Hill Repeats

As the name suggests, these are repetitive "charges," or fast-paced efforts run up hills. Considered a strengthening workout, hill repeats are integrated into your training schedule in the period immediately following the completion of the base-building stage This is the time period when you slowly and careful build weekly mileage levels (with increases no more than 10 percent per week).

Physical Benefits of Hill Repeats

Even if you live in an area with no hills, you can still do hill repeats by finding a highway overpass or bridge with about a 5 percent grade. Speed workouts are very demanding on your legs, and hill repeats are generally run once a week for three to four weeks to improve a runner's leg strength, and as a very important injury prevention measure. Hill repeats are also an excellent means to prepare the cardiovascular system for speed workouts that will follow.

Mental Benefits of Hill Repeats

Besides the benefits derived from strengthening your legs, hill repeats will enhance your mental toughness for workouts and races in locales where the terrain is hilly. While you may never gain an unconditional love for hill training or racing on courses with hills, you will at least face challenging terrain with confidence.

How to Run Hill Repeats

So, how do you do hill repeats? After a warm-up jog of one to one-and-a-half miles (or a minimum of twelve minutes of easy running), assault the hill at 5K effort pace—that's effort, not speed. The idea is to run up the hill as hard as you can while maintaining good running form.

As you reach the end point of the uphill section, generally 100 meters for the novice and up to 200 meters for the experienced runner, your breathing should feel very labored and your legs quite heavy. Turn around and jog (or walk) very easily down the hill and repeat the process again.

Keep in mind that many more injuries arise from running fast downhill (pounding) than from climbing hills at a fast pace. Again, jog or walk very comfortably down the hill, then continue on flat ground for thirty meters or so before turning around for the next repeat.

Depending on your level of experience, the number of repeats will vary. The novice should do no more than four repeats the first week, adding two additional repeats each week for the next three to four weeks. The experienced runner can begin with six repeats and proceed from there. As with any workout, it is important to cool down by jogging at least a mile (or a minimum of ten to twelve minutes).

ESSENTIALS

Uphill running basics:

- Shorten your stride.
- Lean slightly into the hill.
- Keep your head up, focusing on what's just in front of you rather than the top of the hill or incline.
- Maintain a consistent effort up the hill.
- Swing your arms (up and down rather than side to side).
- Stay mentally focused and self-directed, pushing forward until you complete the hill repeat.

Fartlek Workouts

Fartlek is a Swedish word that means "speed play." It is a type of speed work that is unstructured and can be quite spontaneous in nature. Like hill repeats, the fartlek workout is considered a transition type of workout that is infused into one's training program prior to beginning structured speed training. The central purpose of fartlek runs is to prepare a runner for the anaerobic demands that more structured speed workouts and racing provides. In short, the fartlek workout is designed to be a fun and easy way to introduce speed training into your program.

Whereas more structured speed workouts are generally done on a track or an accurately measured course and encompass specified periods and distances of fast-paced running followed by recovery periods, the fartlek workout is quite different. A fartlek workout can be run in a variety of ways featuring various distances and durations run at a fast pace.

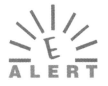

ALERT

Just as fartlek workouts can be run in a variety of ways, these workouts can also be done anywhere, including on roads, trails, and various terrains. Before doing fartleks on hilly courses, it's best to get accustomed to them by running them on flat ground.

Fartlek Running Guidelines

While it is considered an unstructured workout, there are some basic guidelines for fartlek running. Begin your workout with a minimum of one to one-and-a-half miles of easy running (or a minimum of twelve minutes). End with a one-mile cool down, then throw in some speed bursts of varying times and distances each followed by "recovery jogs."

The idea here is to practice running at a brisk effort (generally faster than your present 5K race pace), employing good running form and training your body to run anaerobically (meaning without oxygen). Push yourself until your breathing becomes labored and your pace begins to drop off. Rather than continuing to push yourself at this point (where you are running at a slow pace with deteriorating form due to fatigue), it's much more beneficial to run fast for a shorter period of time and then to resume when you recover (catch your breath).

Planning a Fartlek Workout

In a fartlek workout, some runners will run at a fast pace (at or faster than their current 5K race pace) to a designated landmark such as a telephone pole, then slow down to catch their breath (recover) until they reach the next telephone pole, where they will pick up the pace again. This pattern of running from landmark to landmark is repeated until the conclusion of the workout.

Other runners will plan their fartlek workout to be more specific. For example, after their warm-up period, they will run fast for one minute followed by running a minute at an easy pace to recover. This process could be repeated through the conclusion of the workout. The duration and/or distance of fast-paced running can either be increased or decreased at any time during the workout. The choice is up to you based on your perceived level of effort and the amount of discomfort you wish to experience.

So as not to overdo it and risk incurring an overuse injury, I recommend that you develop a specific plan for incorporating fartlek workouts into your training program. For example, you might want to run thirty seconds fast followed by thirty seconds easy. Then you could throw in a forty-five second burst followed by a forty-five second recovery jog, and so forth.

The first week, the novice might aim for four minutes of total fast-paced running (for example, thirty seconds + thirty seconds + thirty seconds + forty-five seconds + forty-five seconds + thirty seconds + thirty seconds), adding two minutes of fast efforts for each of the next three weeks. By having a specific plan ahead of time for the duration of cumulative fast periods of running you wish to include in the workout, you will be much less likely to become injured by overdoing it.

Striders

Also known as pick-ups, these are generally done following your warm-up jog prior to the beginning of an interval session or road race to get your legs and cardiovascular system prepared for the fast-paced running that will immediately follow. Like a race car driver revving up the engine prior to the beginning of the Daytona 500, striders will get your oxygen and blood flowing at an increased rate so that you can perform optimally.

The distance of striders is approximately eighty meters in length. These are best run on a straightaway rather than around the curves. Begin by gradually increasing your pace so that you're running with a full stride (but not at full speed) by the thirty to forty meters mark. Hold the pace for the next ten meters before gradually reducing your speed to a jog by the end of the eighty meters.

The purpose of the strider is to achieve a long, full stride length at a comfortable speed. You do not want to sprint all out in a strider. Turn around and repeat this process four times for the beginner to ten times for the advanced competitor. Time your striders so that your speed workout or race follows a couple of minutes later.

Tempo Runs

The primary purpose of including tempo runs into your regimen is to increase your anaerobic threshold so that you can maintain a faster pace over longer periods of time. The pace of the tempo run should be about ten to fifteen seconds slower than your present 5K race pace. Depending upon your race goals, the tempo segment of your run can be anywhere from six minutes to twenty minutes or more. When training for longer races such as marathons and half-marathons, tempo runs of thirty minutes and even longer can be done with the fast-paced segments run at approximately your goal race pace.

Rather than doing a structured warm-up that includes stretching and striders, start out your tempo workout by running easily for at least twelve minutes or longer before cruising into the fast segment. An example of a tempo run workout is to run twelve minutes at tempo pace followed by a six-minute recovery jog. You could then tack on another twelve-minute segment at tempo pace before concluding the balance of your workout with easy running.

Races

Besides being a fun way to run at a faster pace, incorporating races into your long-term training program provides several other benefits. Races are a great way to measure your progress and improvement. Races are also a great first step for the beginner to move from a mileage buildup phase to learning to run a bit faster. The novice and experienced runner can use early to mid-season races as tempo workouts.

Regardless of your rationale for including races as part of your training program, it is important to schedule your races based on the following tenant: Allow a day of no racing for each mile raced prior to running your next race. For example, if you are running a 10K (6.2 miles), don't run another 10K race for at least seven days afterwards. You could, however, run a 5K race the following weekend. Similarly, if you run a half-marathon (13.1 miles), don't run another race of any distance within the following fourteen days. Of course, you will need to listen to your body when it comes to running speed workouts within a few days following a race. If your legs feel shot, rest them with easier runs until they feel fresh enough for a hard workout.

Intervals

Interval workouts consist of a series of short, faster paced runs, generally a mile or less in distance, interspersed with recovery jogs. There are many variations of interval workouts, with different rationales behind each. Each has it's own unique benefit. Each type of workout has the long-term goal of improving your overall speed in race distances from the mile to the marathon.

While repeat interval workouts are most often run on a 400-meter track (commonly found on high school and college campuses) they can also be run elsewhere such as on roads and trails. However, should you choose to do these other than on a track, the course/route needs to be measured accurately (to the exact meter) so that the workout is meaningful.

There are three basic types of interval workouts: repeat intervals, pyramids, and ladders. Each will be described below. First, though, some general concepts about intervals need to be introduced.

FACTS

Interval workouts feature two major components. First, they have the fast-paced segment, called the repeat, which is run over a specified distance at a targeted goal time. That is followed by the brief rest period called the recovery.

The theory behind the interval workout is simple. Let's use a 5K (3.1 mile) race for example. Rather than working on improving your speed over the entire 5K distance, it is more effective to run a bit faster than your present race pace over distances shorter than the 5K. Follow these speed intervals with brief periods of rest.

Here's the method. First, you determine your present mile pace at a short distance race such as a 5K. Running this race at a very hard effort gives you important baseline information that you will need to design appropriate speed workouts. The most common interval distances for which to practice fast-pace efforts include 200 meters, 400 meters, 800 meters, 1,200 meters, 1,600 meters, and a mile. There is a myriad of interval workouts that one can run to develop and improve their speed. These will be discussed later in this section. Prior to beginning any type of interval session, it is very important to begin your workout with a thorough warm-up (featuring easy jogging, stretching, and striders). Equally important is the cool-down, which concludes the workout. All of these are described in detail later in this chapter.

There are several variables within an interval workout that one can tweak to vary the level of difficulty. The target time for the interval can be adjusted up or down, the recovery (time or distance) can be increased or decreased, and the number of repeats can be increased or decreased. If you are a novice, an experienced runner or a coach can assist you in designing interval workouts that are appropriate for your present ability level, and your short- and long-term running goals.

The target time for the interval (the fast-paced segment), as mentioned earlier, is usually based on your current race pace at a short race distance such as a 5K. While novices first attempting interval workouts might practice running the shorter segments at their current race pace, more experienced competitors would do these twenty to thirty seconds per mile faster.

For the experienced runner, the recovery jog that follows the repeat is typically half the distance of the interval you ran. The novice first attempting these workouts should allow a longer recovery period. The recovery period can also be expressed as a time that is approximately the same duration as the fast segment previously run.

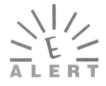

The quality of your interval workout may be affected by leg fatigue resulting from not getting enough rest. Also, you may not have warmed up properly. Perhaps you require a longer warm-up jog or need to stretch a bit more. Environmental conditions such as warm temperatures/high humidity or stiff headwinds also can negatively affect your performance during these fast-paced workouts.

Repeat Intervals

These are workouts where the distance of the fast-paced segment remains constant. For example, the workout could feature six 400-meter repeats with a 200-meter recovery jog after each. Or four 800-meter repeats each followed by a 400-meter recovery jog.

It is important to run consistent times for the repeats. You should try to run the final repeat in approximately the same time as you ran the first. The idea here is to leave the track feeling that if you wanted to, you could do one or two more intervals. If you find that your speed really falls off after the first couple of intervals, your target time for these may be too fast for your current level of conditioning. You can either adjust the workout accordingly from the original plan by increasing your goal times for the repeats (running the repeats at a slower pace), allow yourself more recovery between the fast-paced segments, or bag the workout entirely and attempt it another day.

Abbreviations are often used in books, magazine articles, or by coaches to describe specific speed workouts. For example: 6 × 400M in 1:40, 200R. means that you will be asked to run six 400-meter repeats (once around the track) in one minute and forty seconds, followed by a 200-meter recovery jog after each of the repeats.

Pyramids and Ladders

Pyramids and ladders are also considered to be part of the interval family. Rather than running the same distances for all your intervals, you vary the length of each interval, running longer or shorter intervals throughout the workout. Pyramid workouts feature fast segments increasing and then decreasing in distance. For example, your fast segments could progress upwards with 200, 400, and topping out at 800 meters before going down again to a 400 and 200.

A ladder is a progression either up or down in interval length. For example, your intervals could progress upward with longer and longer lengths: 200 meters, followed by 400, 800, 1,200, and ending with 1,600 meters. Or the ladder workout could be run in the reverse order beginning with your longest distance of your fast-paced segments run first (1,600, 1,200, 800, 400, 200).

Important Warm-up Procedures

With the exception of fartlek and tempo runs (you will be doing some easy jogging prior to rolling into the fast-paced segments of these), it is important to develop a regular thorough warm-up routine that you can utilize for every interval workout and race. The warm-up is important for three reasons. First of all, running at a fast pace without a proper warm-up greatly increases your chances of incurring an injury. Secondly, your muscles will perform more efficiently and optimally after being properly warmed up. Third, you will be following a consistent routine that will decrease high anxiety and stress levels that can sometimes precede difficult workouts and races.

Make Time to Warm Up

It is very important to plan for and allow adequate time for your warm-up so that you're not rushed getting to the starting line of a race. Similarly, you don't want to rush through a warm-up (or cool-down for that matter) so that you won't be late for a personal commitment such as work or dinner with the family.

You want your warm-up routine to be the same each and every time out so that it becomes a regular habit. You want it to feel comfortable so that you are confident that you are prepared both physically as well as mentally for the challenges a speed workout or race provides. As mentioned previously, using the same warm-up routine for races, you will reduce your level of anxiety and nervousness on race day.

Your Warm-up Routine

Begin your warm-up with a minimum of twelve minutes of easy jogging. In situations where you will be racing shorter distances such as the 5K, or when the weather is cold, you may want to increase the time/distance of your warm-up jog. After months and years of experience, you may perhaps find that you will perform better with a longer warm-up.

Next, you want to stretch all your major leg muscles thoroughly (calves, hamstrings, quads, hips) for several minutes. Again, don't rush yourself! While stretching, you may want to take a few swigs of water to top off your reservoir. So as to have an effective speed workout without interruptions, it's better to hydrate at this time. However, if it's a warm day, use common sense and take fluids as often as the conditions dictate. If it is too hot and humid that day, reschedule the workout for another day in the week (however, keeping in mind the hard/easy concept of training mentioned throughout the book).

The last thing to do prior to your speed workout or race is to run four to ten striders of eighty meters, as described above. After completing these, take a minute or two to catch your breath. You are now prepared to run hard.

ESSENTIALS
Rather than running lap after lap on the track (which can be quite boring!) do your warm up on a road or a grass field. Spare your knees, ankles, and hips of unnecessary wear and tear as a result of the frequent turns on the track.

Important Cool-Down Procedures

Don't consider your workout or race over until you cool down properly. Even for your daily runs that are performed at a comfortable pace, you should finish up the workout by jogging easily the last ten minutes and then stretch immediately afterwards.

After running at a fast pace, it is even more important to jog easily for ten minutes or longer so that your breathing and heart rate can return to normal. Following your cool-down jog, invest ten to fifteen minutes into stretching your major leg muscles (along with any upper body parts that feel tight) thoroughly before calling it quits. By cooling down properly, your muscles will recover effectively from the demands of the hard workout or race. Compared to the runner who rushes through or skips his/her cool-down, your muscles will feel much less stiff, sore, and fatigued later in the day. In addition, you will be fully recovered and ready to perform optimally for your next workout.

Speed Work Programs Based on Experience

The most important thing to remember when developing a program integrating advanced training techniques is that there is no "cookie cutter" or "one size fits all" approach. Programs must be individualized to meet your present ability level as well as your goals and needs. This section will provide a wide range of essential guidelines for the runner who is first attempting speed work and for the experienced and accomplished runner.

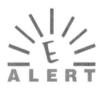

If you are a beginner attempting speed work for the first time, do not jump ahead and attempt workouts designed for the novice or experienced runner. Injury can almost be guaranteed! By the same token, the novice runner should not attempt the experienced runners' workouts. The key point to remember is that progress comes with consistent training over months and years of time. Be patient. Train only at your present ability level!

The Beginner

The beginner is the person who has just started a running program over the past year. As mentioned, the beginner's primary focus should be to build a base where one is running consistently for a year reaching weekly levels of twenty to twenty-five miles per week. By exercising patience during this time, leg muscles will be strengthened to later be able to handle the rigors of more advanced training. Pushing the limits by doing speed workouts at this time before leg muscles have strengthened adequately will greatly increase risk of injury.

Rather than including advanced training techniques into their program, it's perfectly fine for beginners to enter races of 5K and 10K distances once a month or so for fun and to gain the experience provided by running in an organized and competitive forum. By occasionally participating in road races, beginners will gain an understanding of their present ability level (race pace) while learning the value of even pacing.

The Novice

A novice runner is one who has consistently been running twenty to twenty-five miles per week for a year or more. After a base-building phase, novices can add some advanced training techniques into their training schedule.

This phase can begin with four weeks of hill repeats performed one time per week. Novices can start with four repeats up a 5 percent grade of 100 meters long, adding two repeats for each of the next three weeks. Refer to the hill repeat section presented earlier in this chapter for guidelines.

Fartlek runs can then be utilized during the next four weeks as a means of transitioning from the hill repeat phase to interval training. The novice should begin with four minutes of cumulative fast-paced efforts one time per week and increase the duration by two minutes each week for the next three weeks. Please refer to the fartlek section presented earlier in this chapter for additional guidelines.

Following the eight combined weeks of hills and fartlek workouts, novices are now ready to include more structured speed work into their training over the next six weeks. Replace the fartlek workout with some repeat intervals. While there are a myriad of options regarding workouts, one possible plan could be to alternate these weekly speed sessions between 400-meter and 800-meter repeats. For either workout, be sure not to increase the distance of the fast-paced running by more than a total of

800 meters per week. The speed of these repeats should be at their current race pace with an equal amount of recovery jogging as the repeat (fast-paced segment) that was performed.

Every third or fourth week, enter a 5K or 10K race to evaluate your training progress. Determine your race pace by checking the split times at each mile-mark, or calculate your average mile pace from your overall finish time. You can then adjust the speed of future repeat intervals accordingly to allow for continued improvement.

Now is the time to tackle your target race. I recommend that you taper the final week before the race by cutting your weekly mileage in half. Throw in a few thirty-second bursts of speed to top off training during the last speed work session three to four days before the big event. During the race, focus on running an even but aggressive pace that you can maintain throughout the entire race. Turn on the "afterburners" the last 800 meters and try to pass as many runners as possible while maintaining good running form.

The Experienced Runner

The guidelines for base building for the experienced runner are the same as for the beginner and novice. However, the experienced runner may find that he/she performs best with weekly mileage levels at forty to forty-five miles per week. Some advanced competitors log weekly mileage at even significantly higher levels; however, lingering leg fatigue and the increased risks of injury may outweigh the gains of additional mileage run per week. The key point to remember is that more is not always better, also keeping in mind to put an emphasis on quality over quantity.

Many experienced runners can handle two advanced training workouts per week. Assuming that their long run is on Sunday, the advanced runner could do a fartlek workout on either Tuesday or Wednesday followed by a hill repeat workout on either Thursday or Friday the first four weeks of this phase of training. Listening to your body is the best way to determine which days your legs will feel most rested and recovered for these advanced workouts. Please refer to the guidelines provided earlier in this chapter on fartlek and hill repeats for more information.

For the first week, the fartlek workout would encompass six minutes of cumulative fast-paced efforts with four minutes added per session for each of the next three weeks. Similarly, the hill repeats would begin with six charges up a 150-200 meter incline with two repeats added per session for each of the next three weeks.

After completing four weeks of fartlek runs and hill repeats, more formal speed training (interval sessions) can begin and continue over the next eight to ten weeks. Again, assuming that your long run is Sunday, interval sessions could be performed either on Tuesdays or Wednesdays depending on what day your legs feel most rested. How quickly you run these fast segments will be determined by your present 5K race pace.

For the sake of this discussion, let's say that your present race pace is 8:00 per mile. In the first week of interval training, aim to run the 400-meter repeats at 7:40 pace per mile (1:55 per lap) followed by a 200-meter recovery jog. Repeat this sequence three more times, striving to run a consistent pace for each interval. The next week, run 800 meters at 7:50 pace per mile (3:55 for two laps) with a 400-meter recovery jog. Repeat this process two more times.

As your speed improves over the course of your race season, target the 400-meter repeat times to be approximately twenty to twenty-five seconds faster than your current 5K race pace. The 800-meter repeats should be run about ten to fifteen seconds faster than your 5K race pace. By the end of this phase of training, weekly interval sessions will top-out with workouts of ten to twelve 400-meter repeats and five to six 800-meter repeats. Remember that with any speed workout or race, it is very important to include at least a one to one-and-a-half mile warm-up and a one-mile cool-down jog followed by ten to fifteen minutes of stretching.

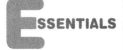
SSENTIALS

The experienced runner can also vary the interval workouts over the course of the next several weeks, beginning with longer repeat intervals during the earlier part of training (1,600 and 1,200 meters) and shortening the fast-paced segments as the target race grows closer. For variety, pyramids and ladder sessions can also be included into the mix of interval session possibilities.

Along with the interval sessions, the experienced runner might also want to include some tempo workouts during this period of training. Tempo runs will provide the opportunity to practice running at a fast pace for longer periods of time. These could be scheduled two to three days following the interval workout session or can occasionally be nested within a ten- to twelve-minute run. The first week, aim to sustain a swift pace for six continuous minutes within the middle part of the workout, adding an additional four minutes for each subsequent week. The pace of the tempo segment should be run approximately ten to fifteen seconds per mile slower than present 5K race pace.

Every third or fourth week, a 5K or 10K practice race can be substituted for a tempo workout/long run to evaluate training progress.

From these practice events, determine your current race pace (per mile) and adjust the speed of future repeat interval sessions accordingly to allow for continued improvement.

After the completion of the interval phase of training, one is now ready to race at his/her optimal level. Through the experience gained over the course of months and years of racing, advanced competitors better understand the maximum level they can push and maintain their race pace. Unlike the beginner and novice, where improvement is often measured in minutes, the experienced runner may only be able to improve by a few seconds from race to race.

ALERT

Reduce the strain on your knees (thus minimizing your risk of injury) when running on the track by changing your running direction midway through your speed workout. Important: Change directions only if no other runners or walkers are using the track. If you are running the workout with a group, make sure that the other runners also agree to do so.

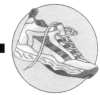

CHAPTER 12

Training and Running a Half-Marathon

The desire to race a half-marathon (13.1 miles) is a natural progression for many runners who have completed a mileage buildup program and wish to undertake new goals. While it doesn't require the same degree of commitment as training for a marathon, the half-marathon is still a worthy challenge that many runners around the world seek.

Mileage Buildup for the Half-Marathon

Begin your half-marathon training by finding the training week/level from one of the two mileage buildup schedules that most closely matches your present training routine (refer to Chapter 5 for these buildup schedules). From that point, proceed until you complete the remaining mileage specified on whichever schedule you have been using.

Next, continue your training by following your choice of the two schedules that are featured below. The maximum distance of your longest training run (and thus choice of charts) will be determined in part by your competitive aspirations along with how much you enjoy doing long runs. The longest training run (sixteen miles) should be completed no more than three weeks before the half-marathon. Run at least twelve miles in practice to be minimally prepared for the 13.1 mile race.

NOVICE HALF-MARATHON TRAINING SCHEDULE

WEEK #	SUN.	MON.	TUE.	WED.	THUR.	FRI.	SAT.	TOTAL
1	11	Rest	5	7	5	Rest	5	33
2	12	Rest	5	7	5	Rest	5	34
3	8	Rest	6	Rest	4	Rest	2	18–20
							Opt.	TAPER WEEK
4	13.1 (RACE DAY)	Rest	4	5	4	Rest	5	31

ADVANCED HALF-MARATHON TRAINING SCHEDULE

WEEK #	SUN.	MON.	TUE.	WED.	THUR.	FRI.	SAT.	TOTAL
1	11	Rest	6	8	5	Rest	5	35
2	12	Rest	6	8	5	Rest	5	36
3	8	Rest	4	6	4	Rest	4	26
								EASY WEEK
4	14	Rest	6	8	6	Rest	5	39
5	16	Rest	6	8	6	Rest	5	41
6	13	Rest	5	7	5	Rest	5	35
7	10	Rest	4	Rest	4	Rest	2	18–20
							Opt.	TAPER WEEK
8	13.1 (RACE DAY)	Rest	4	6	4	Rest	4	31

The Long Run

While the long run is discussed in great detail in the marathon training chapters of this book (Chapters 16 and 17), the key points regarding this important workout are highlighted here. Similar to marathon training, the long run is the most important component of one's half-marathon training because it teaches the body to both mentally and physically tackle the challenges presented in completing races of 13.1 miles and longer. For the purposes of this discussion, the distance of a long run is considered to be ten miles or longer, or a run that lasts more than ninety minutes.

The long run also provides an excellent opportunity to experiment with a variety of issues and concerns, such as shoes, nutrition, or pacing. Above all, long-distance training schedules must be designed so that runners are rested prior to undertaking their long runs. Runners who complete at least two long runs of ten miles prior to a half-marathon will be better prepared to face the challenge ahead of them.

E
ALERT

Don't split your long run! If your training schedule calls for a long run of ten miles, the distance must be run at one time rather than splitting the distance into a five-mile morning session and a five-mile evening run.

Things to Consider While Running Long

The majority of runners who experience difficulty in completing their long training runs fail to prepare adequately for these critical workouts. The following guidelines will enable you to prepare for and complete your long runs safely and successfully. Completing all of your scheduled long runs will in turn greatly enhance your chances of performing well on race day.

Pace and Time

Run at a conversational pace by starting out slowly to conserve glycogen. Your long-run pace should be approximately one to one-and-a-half minutes slower than your present 10K race pace. You should be running so that your perceived exertion level seems easy and relaxed. Put another way, if you wished to carry on a lengthy conversation with another runner, you could easily do so without gasping for air.

There are two major reasons for the need to run at a relaxed pace during the long run. Most importantly, you will be conserving glycogen and glucose (your energy source, converted from digested food that is stored in your working muscles and blood supply, respectively). Running at an easy pace also reduces the possibility of incurring an injury. This is particularly important, as you will probably be building your mileage to levels as yet unachieved. This in itself puts stress and strain on your muscles, joints, tendons, and ligaments.

As you focus on your pace, also consider running for cumulative time, approximating the distance you travel. For example, if your easy-run pace is ten minutes per mile, run for ninety or so minutes for your ten-miler rather than finding a course that is exactly that distance. Doing so will enable you to have more flexibility and spontaneity in regards to the route you choose to run. Schedule some long runs at the same time of day the actual race will be held to familiarize yourself with running during that timeframe and to also develop a pre-race routine that feels comfortable to you.

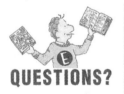

QUESTIONS?

Should I do long runs with others?
For your long runs, either run with friends or find a group running *at your pace.* Running with a group will make the long run more pleasurable and easier to accomplish than running alone.

Running Form and Upper Body Considerations

While there is no need to alter your running stride, you need to focus on keeping your upper body relaxed and loose. Remember, tension is the adversary of all long-distance runners. Tension in the arms, shoulders, and especially the back drains energy and makes running more difficult. It creates stress that takes away from the main focus—running. Shake out your arms and shoulders regularly to combat tension.

Carry your arms close to your waist or hips to conserve energy. Also avoid unnecessary arm swing, particularly laterally across the body. Remember, this is wasted motion and energy expenditure, and it also puts extra strain on your hips.

Hydration

Water and sports drinks are your "lifeline" to completing these long runs. It is very important that you drink fluids every twenty-five to thirty minutes while you are running, regardless of weather conditions. For runs that are more than an hour long, you also need to drink sports drinks such as Gatorade or Powerade to fuel those working muscles, keeping them functioning optimally.

Don't rely on your thirst mechanism to send a signal to your brain saying, "I'm thirsty!" If you wait until that point, you will be not be able to consume enough fluids to catch up with your hydration needs. Doing so puts you at a greater risk of varying degrees of heat illness (check out Chapter 9 for more information on running in the heat). In short, dehydration is one of your biggest enemies. Many beginners fail to grasp this and ignore opportunities to take on fluids. Don't pass these up. Drink!

Psychological Issues

Realize that long runs will sometimes be difficult to complete and that you may experience some "bad patches" in the later miles. Persevering through these stretches will help you to develop mental toughness, a skill that will be essential during a half-marathon or a full marathon. Use imagery, mental rehearsal/visualization, and self talk to develop mental toughness (see Chapter 16). For example, to make the run seem more doable, try to mentally break the course into sections. That is, mentally run from one landmark to the next instead of thinking of completing the entire ten-mile training course. When you reach the first landmark, then mentally think of running to the next, and so forth.

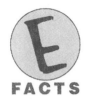

FACTS

The half-marathon is a great race to use as a marathon "tune up." It provides the opportunity to experiment with a variety of factors, such as pre-race routine, nutrition, or pacing. Additionally, one's marathon finish time can be extrapolated somewhat from the half-marathon distance. However, marathon predictor charts have less reliability if one hasn't completed at least two runs of over twenty miles.

Areas of Experimentation

One extremely beneficial aspect of the long run that can't be overlooked is the opportunity to experiment with a variety of miscellaneous concerns, from shoes to foods, prior to incorporating them into long-distance events such as the half-marathon. A cardinal rule of long distance racing is: Don't try anything new or leave anything to chance on race day. Use all training runs as opportunities for experimentation. For a variety of issues for which you should consider experimenting long before race weekend arrives, see the final section of this chapter, "Runners, Take Your Mark, Set, Race!"

When the Long Run Is Over

You mean you have to do something after the run is over? Yes! Sometimes injuries occur as a result of not giving your fatigued muscles the cool down that they need and deserve. Follow these three simple guidelines after every long-distance run and you'll feel better.

Drink and Eat

You've sweated the miles, you've burned off the calories, you've earned it! Of course, this isn't an invitation to pig out and throw all dietary caution to the wind. "Eat, drink, and be merry," as the saying goes, but do so in moderation.

Cool Down

Cool down by running the last half-mile slowly. Or, once you've crossed the finish line, walk for awhile or jog another half-mile to slow your body down. It may sound crazy, but it will work wonders and your body will, in fact, feel better for it.

Stretch

After you've walked a little and had something to drink, stretch thoroughly while your muscles are still warm. This can't be stated strongly enough, as your muscles will probably be tight from the long distance that you've covered. Don't wait until you've cooled off, because if you do, you'll be more likely to hurt yourself. Also, stretching warm muscles will help make them less stiff and painful later on in the day.

ESSENTIALS

You might want to do some other activities after completing your long run and half-marathon. Do some light cycling or walking later in the day to loosen up your legs. You could also consider utilizing therapeutic techniques such as dipping your legs in cool water immediately after the run or getting a leg massage over the next couple of days to reduce muscle soreness and fatigue.

Runners, Take Your Marks, Set, Race!

For the sake of discussion, assume that your half-marathon race is scheduled for Sunday at 8:00 A.M. By practicing/experimenting with these issues and concerns prior to and during your long training runs, you greatly increase the chances that your half-marathon experience will be a successful one.

Rest

First, you need to get lots of rest Saturday night. Aim for at least eight hours of sleep. What you don't want to do is tire out your legs, so make either Friday or Saturday a complete rest day for the legs. If you must train, do something light (not a run). If you train on Saturday, make it a very light workout on the legs.

Nutrition

What you drink and eat can make a big difference to your performance on race day. First, drink lots of water. You have to fight the possibility of dehydration, so drink water all day Saturday. Additionally, you can eat a lot, but make sure you're eating smart. Eat meals high in carbohydrates for lunch and dinner Saturday, but don't eat the wrong foods. Select the "right" pre-race meal for you, such as pasta with marinara sauce as opposed to Alfredo sauce. Avoid foods high in salt and excessive protein or fat all day Saturday. Also, this may surprise you, but go light on salads and vegetables, as these can cause a host of digestive problems.

On Sunday morning, drink about sixteen ounces of water prior to your long run and race. Additionally, eat a light snack Sunday morning before your long run and race. Figure out what and how early you must eat to avoid digestive problems.

While running, you'll want to drink lots of fluids. Be sure to stop for water frequently throughout the run. For runs and races of longer than ninety minutes, you should strive to drink sports beverages every two to three miles or every twenty-five to thirty minutes. Drinking on the run requires careful planning of the route (make sure there is water available frequently, along with places to stash sports drinks). Most races have frequent water stops, and almost all (with the exception of some 5Ks) provide sports drinks.

You may also want to consider using gel carbohydrate replacement products during the run. Be sure to chase them down with water to avoid stomach cramps and to enhance the absorption of these products. (Please dispose of gel and energy wrappers properly by throwing them away in trash receptacles or placing them in your fanny pack. Let's all work together to keep the environment clean! Nothing worse than a disrespectful runner.)

Finally, after the run is over, continue to drink fluids (water, sports drinks, or juice are all great choices). Also eat some more; you've earned it! As soon as possible (ideally within fifteen minutes of the end of the race), have something to eat to replace depleted glycogen stores. Research has shown that to avoid muscle fatigue the next day, carbohydrates should be eaten as soon as possible following long duration exercise.

Shoes, Apparel, and Accessories

You should remember that especially for a long run, good equipment is essential. To get through the long run and race comfortably, pay particular attention to your shoes, apparel, and accessories.

For you footwear, make sure that your shoes have low mileage to maximize absorption of shock. Do not wear new shoes or shoes that are not sufficiently broken in for a long run or race. On the other hand, make sure the shoes you will wear aren't broken down.

In addition to shoes, comfortable and functional clothing is one of the most important ingredients for runs of all distances, but in particular, the long run and races. Wear Coolmax or synthetic blend socks, singlets, shorts, and leggings that wick away moisture and won't cause chafing. Again, don't wear anything for the first time there at the race. Wear socks and other apparel that have at least been worn once during training and that have been washed. With accessories, remember to use Skin-Lube or Vaseline (on feet, under arms, between thighs, nipples, etc.) to eliminate or reduce chafing and/or blisters.

When dressing for a run, remember that excess clothing causes overheating of the body. Once you begin running, it will feel as if ten degrees has been added to the outside temperature. Also remember that hats will trap body heat, making them great for a cold weather race but a bad idea for a race with hot/humid conditions.

CHAPTER 13
Injury Prevention

The majority of running injuries occur from training errors. To avoid injury, your increase in mileage and speed should be gradual. It is important to intersperse hard days and easy days, as well as hard and easy weeks. Mileage should be increased approximately 10 percent per week, and every fourth week you should back off slightly.

Avoiding Injury: The Basics

For most runners, at least one or two days a week should be devoted to rest or non-running activities. This gives your body a chance to recover and strengthen itself. It is also helpful to maintain a running diary, which should contain your mileage, course, and brief note on how you felt during each run. Such a record may help trace the origin of any number of training errors.

As you progress in your running program, you should always ease into speed work. Following a gradual and consistent mileage buildup period, some ways to ease into speed work might be throwing in a few short-distance surges into your normal runs, hill work, and fartlek runs. Track workouts should occur after you have accomplished some faster-paced running during the course of your routine runs and should not be overly ambitious at first. (See Chapter 10 for a thorough discussion of the precautions that need to be taken prior to including faster-paced workouts into your training.)

A Look at Athletic Shoes

Running shoes should be replaced regularly. The shock-absorbing capability of the midsole will diminish gradually and may be inadequate after 350 to 500 miles. The number of miles depends upon a variety of factors that may include, among others, the runner's weight, training terrain, and environmental conditions. The upper of the shoe may not show much wear, but the shock absorption may already be gone. If you are running approximately twenty miles per week, you should be replacing your shoes between four and six months, depending upon your shock absorption needs.

Problems Related to Running Shoe Design Flaws

Even if you are a careful runner, stretching consistently and not overextending yourself in your runs, you can incur injury from running in poorly designed shoes. By recognizing the potential problems associated with faulty shoe design, you can become a more discerning shoe buyer and ensure that the shoes you are wearing meet your biomechanical needs.

Achilles Tendonitis

Shoes that have inflexible soles cause the calf muscles to work harder and can contribute to the development of Achilles tendonitis, in which the Achilles tendon becomes inflamed. The mechanical reason for this is best explained by looking at the foot as a fulcrum and lever system. Shoes with inflexible soles make the lever arm (the foot) function over a longer distance and make the tip of the shoe the location of the fulcrum (the pivot point). Ideally, the shoe should flex at the point where the toes join the foot, which also happens to be the widest part of the shoe, offering more support. The shoe should also have a slight heel lift, which most running shoes do.

Shoes that have too much heel cushioning, including some of the air-cushioned models, can also contribute to Achilles tendonitis. After the heel strikes the ground, it continues moving, as the shoe's cushioning continues to absorb shock. This continued motion can stretch a susceptible Achilles tendon excessively.

Plantar Fasciitis

Shoes that are too flexible in the mid-sole or that flex before the point at which the toes join the foot result in forces that can both directly cause a stretch in the *plantar fascia* (the bowstring-like tissue on the sole of your foot) and contribute to excess pronation in the foot. The lack of stability that exists in a shoe with this characteristic occurs not just at the transverse plane of the shoe where the shoe actually flexes, but also in a longitudinal plane, reducing the effectiveness of the shoe in controlling pronation.

Tips for Buying and Wearing Shoes

A shoe's mid-sole only lasts so long. It degrades from use, and the resultant useful life of a running shoe is 350 to 500 maximum miles. This means that if you are running about twenty miles a week, you should consider changing shoes at weeks twenty to twenty-five. Although the shoes may no longer be good for running, they may still serve a useful purpose, such as casual wear for walking.

When assessing the condition of your running shoes, realize that sole wear does not necessarily reflect the loss of shock absorption by a shoe. Even a new-looking shoe may lack adequate shock absorption. Use the 350 to 500 mile guideline instead of trying to guess how worn your shoe should look.

When buying your running shoes, make sure there is about a thumb's width at the front of the shoe. This will help prevent runner's (black) toe and/or loosing one's toenails. The shape and depth of the front of the shoe also have an effect on these problems.

If you have had no problems while running in a shoe, you should probably buy another pair of the same make and model. Should that style/model be discontinued by the manufacturer (a very common occurrence!), see if it's available through a running specialty store or look at ads in the back of a magazine like *Runner's World*.

Make sure you carefully lace your shoe before running. Too tight a shoe may make parts of the top of your foot sore or squeeze your metatarsals too tightly. This in turn can result in the feelings of numbness and/or tingling in one's feet, particularly on long training runs. Too loose a shoe may make your foot move excessively and be less stable, resulting in more than normal pronation, also increasing the possibility of blisters.

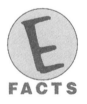

FACTS

Don't even dream of running a marathon in a new pair of shoes. Your shoes should have at least seventy miles, which includes one long training run of twenty miles or longer, to be broken in well enough to run a marathon.

Shoe Wear: What Can It Tell You?

Shoe wear is often believed to hold much meaning. However, while shoe wear may tell you much, there is much ambiguity present as well. Although some would disagree, more conclusive evidence can be found by examining the foot and observing gait. This can tell a doctor more about how your shoes will wear than examining your shoes will tell you about either your feet or your gait.

With that said, there are some things you can learn from looking at shoe wear. One is asymmetry in wear. This will reflect asymmetry of function. There may be a leg length difference, one foot may pronate more than the other, muscles may be tighter or weaker on one side, or a rotational deformity may be present.

Rearfoot Strikers

If there is wear on the outer heel of your running shoe, you may be a rearfoot striker. The point of initial contact with the ground is usually the place showing the most wear. Of course, this could be normal wear, as most people have wear here. This can occur with a slight outtoe (toes point the feet outward rather than straight ahead) and the increase in the varus foot position that occurs in running because of the narrower base of gait (the distance from the midline that the foot strikes the ground).

Wear on the inner heel indicates a rearfoot striker. You may possibly have an intoe gait (toes point the feet inward rather than straight ahead), which would make this area the initial point of contact with the ground. Inner heel wear could also signify severe pronation, if the heel counter is bent inward and the medial part of much of the sole shows wear. The best way to tell is by really looking at the foot in addition to the shoe.

Forefoot Strikers

Meanwhile, much forefoot wear and little heel wear usually indicates forefoot strike, which the shoes of many faster short- and middle-distance runners will show. Uneven wear, or wear below a second or third metatarsal area may indicate a Morton's foot (short first metatarsal) and excess pronation. The indicated metatarsal may be at higher risk for a stress fracture.

High Arches and Supinating Feet

On the other hand, middle of the sole wear may in general reflect a high arch or excessively supinating foot. Supination is defined as a condition when the feet point outward upon landing (a pigeon-toed footstrike). Medial sole wear, with a bent counter and a medial shift of the upper, probably indicates severe excessive pronation. Additionally, the heel counter may be bent inward with excessive pronation and tilted to the outside by a high arched foot.

The upper may likewise tilt inward with a hyperpronating foot and tilt outward with a supinated (underpronating) foot. It may exhibit holes by the toes, or by the big toe alone. This means it may be too shallow or too short at the front of the foot. There should be a thumb's width at the front of the shoe in front of the toes. If the toes make a big bump in the shoe less than one-half inch from the tip of the shoe, the shoe is probably too short.

Guide to Shoes and Foot-Related Problems

The following are some basics to keep in mind regarding shoe characteristics that will help certain foot problems:

- **Low arch:** This condition needs much support, so choose a stable shoe with good rearfoot control.
- **High arch:** This problem needs more shock absorption, meaning you will do better with a narrower heel.
- **Normal foot:** This is ideal, so you'll probably do best with a shoe that combines control and shock absorption.
- **Post-stress fracture:** A fracture requires that you don't forget to change your shoes frequently (350 to 400 miles) and get a shoe with adequate shock absorption.
- **Achilles tendinitis:** Tendinitis will necessitate avoiding air soles and excessively spongy heels, using a heel lift, and avoiding shoes that are too stiff in the sole.

Stretching to Prevent Injuries

Stretching is discussed at length in Chapter 7, but it cannot be overemphasized as an injury-preventive routine. Runners frequently develop tightness in the posterior muscle groups. This includes the hamstrings and the calf muscles. The quadriceps and anterior shin muscles may become relatively weak due to muscular imbalance. The abdominal muscles also tend to be weak on runners who do not exercise them.

The Magic Six, Plus Two

George Sheehan recommended a revised set of his "magic six" stretches in several of his columns and in his book *Running to Win* (Rodale Press, 1991). Here is a slightly modified version of Dr. Sheehan's Magic Six:

First, the wall pushup is a calf stretch that stretches one leg at a time. Stand with the rear foot approximately two to three feet from the wall. The rear leg should be straight, the front leg is bent and your hands touch the wall. Feet point straight ahead, heels are on the ground. Hold for thirty seconds, switch legs.

Next is the hamstring stretch: Straighten one leg, place it, with the knee locked, on a foot stool. Bend your body and bring your head towards the leg. Hold this position for thirty seconds and switch sides.

In addition to the hamstring stretch, you can also try the knee clasp. Lie on a firm surface (a carpeted floor or grass is best). Bring both knees to your chest and hold for thirty seconds. This stretches the hamstrings and lower back.

Another excellent stretch is the chest pushup: Lie face down on the floor with your abdomen pressed flat on to the floor. Place your hands flat on the floor, beneath your shoulders. Push your chest up with your arms and hold for thirty seconds.

To do the backward stretch, you simply place the palms of your hands against the small of your back while standing straight. Tighten your buttocks and bend backwards. Hold for thirty seconds.

Meanwhile, the shin splinter is a stretch used to strengthen the shins. To do this, sit on a table with your legs dangling over the side. Place a three to five pound weight over your toes. Flex your foot at the ankle (bend it up). Hold for six seconds, repeat five times.

To strengthen the quadriceps, you can use straight leg lifts. Lying on the floor, flex one knee to approximately a right angle. Lift the other leg rapidly to between thirty and sixty degrees. Lower and repeat ten times. Switch legs, repeat five times, and work up to ten sets of ten repetitions.

Finally, the bent leg sit-up strengthens the abdominals. Dr. Sheehan recommended that the sit up be a gradual one rather than a rapid thrust forward. It should feel as if you are moving forward one vertebra at a time. Lie on the floor with your knees bent. Come forward to a position thirty degrees from the floor. Lie back and then repeat twenty times.

ESSENTIALS

Since almost no runner will perform eight exercises, even if disguised as six plus two, here are the four exercises you really should do for optimal health and injury prevention. One other has been included for those with "runner's knee." The four stretches are: wall pushup, hamstring stretch, knee clasp, and bent leg sit-up. Do straight leg lifts if you have runner's knee.

Overstretching

While many runners neglect stretching, some may overstretch. Surveys of runners have shown that there seem to be two types of runners who have reported more injuries than others. Those who do not stretch very much and those who spend an inordinate amount of time stretching both seem to have significantly more injuries. However, this is not necessarily a causal relationship. Those spending much longer than their peers stretching and who report many injuries might be stretching in response to their injuries. But then again, too much of a good thing might not be good.

Preventing Further Injury

If you are currently injured, now is probably not a great time to start stretching. If your Achilles tendon is sore, don't start on a high-intensity stretching program to try to improve it. You may end up contributing to the statistics that demonstrate that Achilles tendonitis is frequently a long-lasting, chronic problem.

The reason you should not start stretching with an acutely sore body part is that your stretching will probably contribute to continuing to tear the muscle or tendon fibers during the stretching. One of the signs of this will be an increase in pain following your stretching. Let the darn thing heal a bit before trying to stretch it!

First, use a heel lift, avoid hills, decrease your stride, and discard any shoes with any gaseous substance used for shock absorption in the heel. Decrease the intensity and duration of your training runs. Once you are feeling better, probably in about three to six weeks, you can begin a light and easy stretching regimen. A similar rationale may be applied to other body parts that are injured.

The Gait Biomechanics of Foot and Leg Problems

To understand lower extremity problems runners encounter, you should be aware of how biomechanical abnormalities in the lower body are related to specific foot and leg problems. The following is a review of the gait cycle, starting simply and then proceeding to a more complex discussion of foot and lower extremity biomechanics. From there, you will review an outline of a general approach to the lower extremity examination as it pertains to mechanically caused foot and leg problems.

Many specific foot problems are caused by biomechanical faults within the foot or lower extremity. In order to understand the cause of these problems, one must understand the normal anatomy, function, and biomechanics of the lower extremity. It is important to be able to visualize the events of the normal gait cycle during walking or running. The gait cycle can be divided into different phases and subphases, so that each action of the foot and leg can be evaluated at specific sequential time periods.

Anatomy of the Gait

Before understanding the specifics of gait, you must first take a quick look at the bones involved. The key bone structures are the talus and calcaneus (located at the ankle and comprising the subtalar joint), and the navicular and cuboid (located just anterior to these bones). The talus and navicular, along with the calcaneus and cuboid, make up what is known as the mid-tarsal joint. The leg bones of significance include the femur (the thigh bone) and the tibia (the larger of the two lower leg bones). The fibula is the smaller leg bone. In front of the tibia is the patella or kneecap.

Phases of Gait

The gait cycle of each leg is divided into the stance phase and the swing phase. The stance phase is the period of time during which the foot is in contact with the ground. The swing phase is the period of time in which the foot is off the ground and swinging forward.

In walking, the stance phase comprises approximately 60 percent of the gait cycle and the swing phase about 40 percent. The proportion of swing to stance phase changes as the speed of walking or running increases. As the speed is increased, the percentage of time spent in the stance phase decreases. Increased time is then spent in the swing phase, and there is an increase in the importance of swing phase muscles. An important point to note is that in running, an added subphase is present called float phase. During float phase, neither foot is on the ground.

Stance and Swing Phases

While walking, 60 percent of the complete gait cycle is spent in stance phase compared to only 40 percent of the time during running. The time period during which the forces are applied is also dramatically different between running and walking. A walker moving at a comfortable speed of 120 steps per minute has a total cycle time of 1 second. A runner moving at 12 miles per hour has a cycle time of 0.6 second. However, the stance phase has decreased from .62 second to 0.2 seconds.

The stance phase can further be subdivided into its three component phases. The first portion of the stance phase is contact. This phase begins with the contact of the heel to the ground and is completed when the remainder of the foot touches the ground. During this portion of the stance phase, the foot is pronating at the subtalar joint. The leg is internally rotating and the foot is absorbing shock and functioning as a mobile adaptor to the ground surface.

The next portion of the stance phase is called midstance. Midstance phase begins when the entire foot has contacted the ground. The body weight is passing over the foot as the tibia and the rest of the body are moving forward. The opposite leg is off the ground and the foot, in this phase, is bearing body weight alone. During this portion of the stance phase the leg is externally rotating and the foot is supinating at the subtalar joint. It is undergoing a change from being a mobile adaptor to becoming a rigid lever in order to propel the body forward during the final portion of the stance phase, propulsion.

Propulsion begins after heel off and ends with toe off. This phase constitutes the final 35 percent of stance phase. The body is propelled forward during this phase as weight is shifted to the opposite foot as it makes ground contact. The subtalar joint must be in a supinated position in order for this phase to be normal and efficient. If abnormal pronation is occurring, the midstance phase and this phase will probably be prolonged and weight transfer through the forefoot will not be normal.

The swing phase begins immediately after toe off. The first portion of the swing phase is the forward swing, which occurs as the foot is being carried forward. The knee is flexed and the foot is flexed at this time. The next segment of the swing phase is foot descent as the foot is being positioned in preparation for weight bearing and the muscles are stabilizing the body to absorb the shock of heel contact. At heel contact the swing phase ends and a new gait cycle begins.

In normal walking, the foot initially contacts at the heel. The major determinant of where maximum heel wear occurs is the initial point of contact as determined by the transverse plane position of the foot at the time of contact. Medial heel wear is usually an indication of intoeing gait, and usually points to rotational abnormality in the limb above.

In the gait of much faster speeds there may be no initial heel contact. An individual may contact at the midfoot and then rock backwards onto the heel or not touch the heel down at all. An example of this gait pattern would be a sprinter.

Following an understanding of the basic phases of gait, one can proceed to recognizing the motions that occur in the legs and feet and understand the interrelationships of these structures. The period of double support, during which both feet are on the ground, occurs during two time periods in the stance phase, during the initial and final 20 percent of the stance phase.

The terminal double support phase has implications for the final portion of stance phase—the propulsion phase. The propulsive phase may be divided into active and passive phases. The active portion occurs after heel off and before the opposite foot touches down and terminal double support begins. The passive portion of terminal double support begins with the touchdown of the opposite foot. During this passive portion, the foot rapidly unloads. Some people call this subphase pre-swing phase.

At heel contact, the pelvis is in slight external rotation. Slightly after heel contact, as the foot is adapting to the ground, the pelvis rotates internally. Just before toe off, it rotates externally, where it remains during the swing phase.

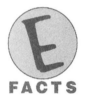

FACTS

During running, if a runner swings his arms across his body, there is a compensatory increase in pelvic rotation. It is more efficient and better for the pelvis and pelvic musculature if the runner moves his arms parallel to the motion in which he is running.

Force Flow

Force flow through the foot may be measured today by a variety of means. The Electrodynogram was the first system available for office use and consisted of seven sensors applied in standard positions on the foot. Other technology accomplishing this exists today. This technology lets us observe forces beneath the foot that normally cannot be seen. It also measures the timing of the phases and subphases of gait and greatly increases the knowledge of what is occurring during the gait cycle. Normal pressure flow through the foot starts slightly lateral in the heel and flows forward to between the first and second metatarsi and exits through the great toe.

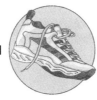

CHAPTER 14

Injury Diagnosis and Treatment

I t is beyond the scope of this book to
discuss in detail the nature and treatment of most running injuries. It is
also difficult to provide detailed information about the treatment of specific injuries
without knowing the symptoms. However,
included in this chapter are some helpful
pointers to consider when you think you
may be injured.

General Guidelines

Should you run with an injury? Perhaps, as long as you can run at a level of intensity below the threshold of pain without altering your normal running stride. When an injury occurs, reduce your mileage and intensity until you can resume running without pain. However, do not take medications or ice an injury before testing whether or not you can run.

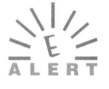

If something hurts, do not run; instead, choose a cross-training activity to maintain cardiovascular fitness. The following sports are generally safe for injured runners: walking, elliptical training, cycling, swimming, deep-water running, rowing, Stair Master, and cross-country ski machines. If you must stop running altogether for more than a week, ease back into your running slowly.

Recognize the difference between fatigue and pain due to an injury. Unfortunately, endorphins (the chemicals the body produces from aerobic exercise) mask pain. Listen to your body and respect what it is telling you.

Some minor discomforts go away once the muscles warm up. Be very cautious in this situation, as you don't want to cause more serious damage to the injury site. Above all, if pain becomes more intense while running, do not continue. Instead, walk and begin treatment.

Inflammation Treatment

Inflammation (characterized by pain, swelling, redness, and warmth) is often the byproduct of many injuries. If inflammation occurs in an injury site, treat the area with ice (see icing guidelines below). Above all, do not treat the area with heat of any kind, wet or dry, for several days.

Consider taking several days off from running along with other types of sports that cause shock to the injured area. Try using some anti-inflammatory medication (such as ibuprofen) for injuries that are inflamed. Be careful not to take too much of these products, as they can cause a variety of internal problems. Heat is a good therapeutic/relaxation measure after inflammation of the injury site has been reduced significantly or eliminated.

If you try all these things and they fail, consider visiting a physician who is familiar with sports injuries and has experience treating runners for both an assessment of the injury and treatment advice. The most important information a physician can provide is whether you can or should continue to run without modification of your training schedule; continue to run with a reduced workload; rest the injury site (e.g., no running); and/or add some cross-training activities to both maintain cardiovascular fitness and to strengthen the injury site.

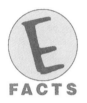

FACTS

To properly ice an injury, use an ice cup. Fill a paper cup with water and then place it in the freezer. When completely frozen, the top of the paper cup can be peeled away to expose the ice. Massage the injured area with the ice cup for approximately ten minutes or until the area is numb. Ice the area again two to three hours later (or as often as possible).

Achilles Tendonitis

Achilles tendonitis is the bane of many runners. The Achilles tendon is what connects the heel and the most powerful muscle group in the body. The Achilles tendon joins three muscles: the two heads of the gastrocnemius and the soleus. The gastrocnemius heads arise from the posterior portions of the femoral condyles. The soleus arises from the posterior aspect of the tibia and fibula.

The gastrocnemius is a muscle that crosses three joints: the knee, the ankle, and the subtalar joint. The functioning of these joints and influence of other muscles on these joints has a significant effect on the tension that occurs within the Achilles tendon. For example, tight hamstrings impact the functioning of the ankle joint, the subtalar joint, and increase tension in the Achilles tendon. The soleus on the other hand does not cross the knee.

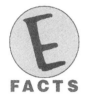

FACTS

The Achilles tendon does not have a rich blood supply. It is not invested within a true tendon sheath; therefore, the blood supply to the proximal portion of the tendon comes from the branches of the muscles themselves.

What Causes Achilles Tendonitis

There are several factors that can contribute to Achilles tendonitis. The biggest contributor to chronic Achilles tendonitis is ignoring pain in your Achilles tendon and continuing to run. If your Achilles tendon is getting sore you should immediately attend to it.

Sudden increases in training can contribute to Achilles tendonitis. Excessive hill running or a sudden addition of hills and speed work can also contribute to this problem.

Two shoe sole construction flaws can also aggravate Achilles tendonitis. The first is a sole that is too stiff, especially at the ball of the foot. If this area is stiff, then the "lever arm" of the foot is longer and the Achilles tendon will be under increased tension, forcing the calf muscles to work harder to lift the heel off the ground.

The second shoe design factor that can lead to a continuing Achilles tendon problem is excessive heel cushioning. Air-filled heels, which supposedly are now more resistant to deformation and leaks, are not good for a sore Achilles tendon. The reason for this is quite simple. If you are wearing a shoe that is designed to give great heel shock absorption, what frequently happens is that after heel contact, the heel continues to sink lower while the shoe is absorbing the shock. This further stretches the Achilles tendon at a time when the leg and body are moving forward over the foot. Change your shoes to one without this feature.

Of course another major factor is excessive tightness of the posterior leg muscles—the calf muscles and the hamstrings—which can contribute to prolonged Achilles tendonitis. Gentle calf stretching should be performed as a preventative measure. During a bout of acute Achilles tendonitis, however, overly exuberant stretching should not be performed.

Treating Achilles Tendonitis

If you are suffering from Achilles tendonitis, the first thing to do is to cut back your training. If you are working out twice a day, change to once a day and take one or two days off per week. If you are working out every day, cut back to every other day and decrease your mileage. Training modification is essential to treatment of this potentially long-lasting problem.

You should also cut back on hill work and speed work. Applying ice after running may also help. Be sure to avoid excessive stretching. The first phase of healing should be accompanied by relative rest, which doesn't necessarily mean stopping running, just a cut back in training. If this does not help quickly, consider having a quarter-inch heel lift put into your shoe. Do not worry that you will become dependent on this; instead, concentrate on getting rid of the pain. Don't walk barefoot around your house and avoid excessively flat shoes, such as sneakers, tennis shoes, cross trainers, and so on.

In-office treatment of Achilles tendonitis would initially consist of the use of the physical therapy modalities of electrical stimulation (HVGS—high voltage galvanic stimulation) and ultrasound. Your sports medicine physician should also carefully check your shoes. A heel lift can also be used, and control of excessive pronation by taping can also be incorporated into a program of Achilles tendonitis rehabilitation therapy. Orthotics with a small heel lift are often helpful.

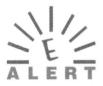

Excessive stretching is not good for your Achilles tendon. In most cases, stretches put too much tension on the already tender Achilles tendon. A wall stretch is a good exception (see Chapter 13).

Achilles Tendon Ruptures

What actually causes the Achilles tendon to rupture is not known. The mechanism of injury is a force that increases the tension in the tendon beyond its tensile strength. A forceful stretch of the tendon or a contraction of the muscles may create this force. Most often it is a combination of the two forces.

Occasionally, ruptures occur at the tendon-bone interface. Since vascularity decreases with age, this frequently occurs in older athletes. A weakening of the Achilles tendon has been observed following intratendinous steroid injection. Therefore, injections of steroids are not recommended at this location. Diseases associated with a possibly increased incidence of tendon rupture include gout, systemic lupus erythematosis, rheumatoid arthritis, and tuberculosis.

Diagnosing a Ruptured Achilles

Physical examination of the site of a recent rupture may reveal a noticeable gap at the site of the rupture. Swelling will be seen. The most frequently described clinical test is called the Thompson test. With the patient lying on his or her stomach, the calf is squeezed. The foot will plantar flex (raise the heel) in a patient who does not have a completely torn Achilles tendon. The foot will not plantar flex when the Achilles tendon is completely torn. An MRI will accurately reveal the extent of the tear. Diagnostic ultrasound is also used to assist in the diagnosis of a torn Achilles tendon.

Treating a Ruptured Achilles Tendon

Complete tears of the Achilles tendon are usually treated with surgical repair followed by up to twelve weeks in a series of casts. Partial tears are sometimes treated with casting for up to twelve weeks alone, and sometimes are treated as complete tears, with surgery and casting. A heel lift is usually used for six months to one year following removal of the cast. Rehabilitation to regain flexibility and then to regain muscle strength are also instituted following removal of the cast.

Runner's Knee

The knee is a complex joint. It includes the articulation between the tibia and femur (leg and thigh) and the patella (kneecap). The most common knee problems in running relate to what is called the "patello-femoral complex." This is the quadriceps, kneecap, and patellar tendon. What is called runner's knee (technically called Chondromalacia Patella Syndrome) is a condition known to the medical community as chondromalacia of the patella, which essentially means softening of the cartilage of the kneecap. Cartilage does not have the same blood supply that bone does. Cartilage relies on intermittent compression to squeeze out waste products and then allow nutrients to enter the cartilage from the synovial fluid of the joint.

Causes of Runner's Knee

During running, certain mechanical conditions may predispose you to a mistracking kneecap. Portions of the cartilage may then be under either too much or too little pressure, and the appropriate intermittent compression that is needed for waste removal and nutrition supply may not be present. This may result in cartilage deterioration, which at the knee usually occurs on the medial aspect or inner part of the kneecap.

The symptoms of runner's knee include pain near the kneecap usually at the medial (inner) portion and below it. Pain is usually also felt after sitting for a long period of time with the knees bent. Running downhill and sometimes even walking down stairs can be followed by pain. When the knee is bent there is increased pressure between the joint surface of the kneecap and the femur (thigh bone). This stresses the injured area and leads to pain.

Factors that increase what is known as the "Q" (quadriceps) angle increases the chance of having runner's knee. The Q angle is an estimate of the effective angle at which the quadriceps averages its pull. It is determined by drawing a line from the anterior superior iliac spine (the bump above and in front of your hip joint) to the center of your kneecap, and a second line from the center of your kneecap to the insertion of the patellar tendon (where the tendon below your kneecap inserts). Normal is below twelve degrees, while definitely abnormal is above fifteen degrees.

Many times adding to the strong lateral pull of the bulk of the quadriceps is a weak *vastus medialis*. This is the portion of the quadriceps that helps medially stabilize the patella. It runs along the inside portion of the thigh bone to join at the kneecap with the other three muscles making up the quadriceps. Some of the mechanical conditions that may contribute to this include:

- Wide hips (female runners)
- Knock knees
- Unstable kneecap (sublaxating patella)
- High kneecap (*patella alta*)
- Small medial pole of patella or corresponding portion of femur
- Weak thigh muscle (*vastus medialis*)
- Pronation of the feet

Treating Runner's Knee

At an early stage of runner's knee, running should be decreased to lessen stress to this area and allow healing to begin. It is important to avoid downhill running, which stresses the patello-femoral complex. Exercises performed with the knee bent should be avoided. When the knee is bent, the forces under the kneecap are increased. Many people feel that the *vastus medialis* muscle works only during the final thirty degrees of extension of the knee. This is the muscle that helps stabilize the kneecap medially and prevents it from shifting laterally and tracking improperly at the patello-femoral joint.

Straight leg lifts strengthen the *vastus medialis* and do not significantly stress the undersurface of the kneecap. They should be done ten times on each side. Start with five sets of ten and work your way up to ten sets of ten. Straight leg lifts are best performed lying on a cushioned but firm surface, with the exercising leg held straight and the non-exercising leg somewhat bent to take pressure off of the back.

Tight posterior muscles should be stretched. In many cases tight calf muscles or hamstrings lead to a "functional equinous" and make the foot pronate while running or walking. This pronation is accompanied by an internal rotation of the leg, which increases the Q angle and contributes to the lateral subluxation of the kneecap. Running shoes that offer extra support should be used. If further control of pronation is needed, orthotics should be considered.

FACTS

The late George Sheehan, M.D., sports medicine physician and philosopher, was the first to popularize the notion that it was important to look at the foot when runner's knee occurs. It is also important to rule out other knee problems when knee pain occurs in runners and not just lump every pain as "runner's knee."

Iliotibial Band (ITB) Syndrome

Symptoms of the iliotibial band syndrome are pain or aching on the outer side of the knee. This usually happens in the middle or at the end of a run. Factors contributing to this syndrome are *genu varum* (bow legs), pronation of the foot (subtalar joint pronation), leg length discrepancy, and running on a crowned surface. Circular track running may also contribute to this problem, since it stresses the body in a manner similar to that of crowned surfaces and leg length differences.

Anatomy of the IT Band

All of these factors are aggravated by a tight iliotibial band. The iliotibial band is a thickening of the lateral (outer) soft tissue that envelops the leg, which is called the fascia. In this area it is called the *fascia lata*. The thickened band is called the iliotibial band. Changes in training (often sudden increases in mileage) frequently contribute to this problem. It is always important to examine your training regimen and see what alterations have recently occurred.

Treatment for ITB Syndrome

To self-treat this problem, you should:

- Temporarily decrease training
- Side stretch
- Avoid crowned surfaces or too much running around a track
- Shorten your stride
- Wear more motion control shoes to limit pronation
- Carefully examine your training regimen (and running diary)

Side stretching is performed while standing as follows: Place the injured leg behind the good one. If the left side is the sore side, cross your left leg behind your right one. Then lean away from the injured side towards your right side. Lean on a table or chair for balance as you do this. Hold for seven to ten seconds and repeat on each side seven to ten times. Be careful not to overstretch.

ESSENTIALS If your self-treatment has not been completely successful, then a trip to a sports medicine specialist may include the additional treatment of either a steroid injection below the IT band and a recommendation for orthotics. Treatment is usually successful for this problem.

Athlete's Foot

You don't have to be an athlete to have athlete's foot. The condition got its name because it is spread in warm moist places, such as locker rooms. Athlete's foot is also known as *tinea pedis*. *Tinea* is from a Latin word that means maggot or grub, and *pedis* refers to the foot. Athlete's foot is actually caused by a fungus or a type of mold and less often by a yeast. Fungus flourishes in dark, warm, moist environments. Shoes, being an occlusive covering of the foot, can be like a fungal heaven.

Clinical Appearance of Athlete's Foot

Athlete's foot can appear as cracked and peeling skin between the toes or on the bottom of the foot. It is often itchy, but not always. Sometimes one only sees flaking, scaling, dry skin that most people think is just a bit of excessive dryness but in reality is evidence of athlete's foot. Small blisters may occur in conjunction with some fungal infections.

Between the toes the skin can become macerated or excessively soft and mushy. The fungus can go deeper into the skin, and through cracks or breaks in the skin bacteria can enter and cause a more troubling secondary bacterial infection.

Preventing Athlete's Foot

As with many things, the best cure is prevention, so we will start with an approach to limiting your risks of contracting athlete's foot. Since moisture is a risk factor, keeping your feet dry is important. Make sure you dry your feet carefully after showers. In the locker room, you might consider wearing shower sandals to limit exposure to any areas contaminated with fungus. Be careful to dry between your toes and make sure your feet are dry before putting on your socks. You may sprinkle an anti-fungal foot powder in your shoes or on your feet.

Another important thing to remember is that cotton socks hold moisture against the foot and do not allow the moisture to readily evaporate. Athletes performing endurance sports should make sure that they wear socks that are made of non-cotton material that wicks the moisture away from the foot.

Treating Athlete's Foot

Mild fungal infections may be treated with over-the-counter medicine that is readily found in your pharmacy. Stubborn fungal infections will require prescription strength medicine. Make certain that you follow the directions for prevention to avoid a recurrence and to speed up elimination of the fungal infection. Keeping your feet dry is one of the keys to eliminating and preventing reinfection.

Side Stitches

Side stitches are pains that occur usually just under the ribs when running. It seems that an unconditioned diaphragm is the cause of this pain more often than not. Some other causes for this pain include food allergies (often milk), gas, or just having eaten before running. Also, running a greater distance than usual or at a faster pace than usual will bring this on. Side stitches seem to occur most often on the right side of the body. It is possible that the liver may alter the motion of the diaphragm more on that side because of the larger right lobe.

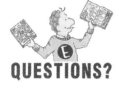

QUESTIONS?

What is a diaphragm?
The diaphragm is a muscle that separates the chest cavity from the abdomen. It moves down when you inhale and moves up when you exhale. When it is subject to more or faster exercise than it is accustomed to it can "cramp" and cause pain.

When caused by lack of conditioning, the best thing to do for side stitches is to run slower and longer. Breathe fuller and try "belly breathing," where you allow your stomach to be "relaxed" and pushed out as you inhale and then contracted slightly as you exhale fully. Breathe rhythmically and make sure that you are not holding your breath. You can also try counting your breaths (six in, hold, three out with a forceful exhalation for a four-count) or whatever seems to work best for you and your running rhythm.

Another breathing tactic is exhaling against resistance through pursed lips. This, combined with belly breathing, may be the best approach. To further strengthen your diaphragm, add abdominal exercises to your regimen.

Dry Heaves or Vomiting

Dry heaves have been associated with training that goes into the anaerobic (without oxygen) realm, and a buildup of lactic acid used to be considered one of its causes.

Some coaches would reportedly keep a bucket at the side of the track for runners who threw up or had the dry heaves. Those coaches felt that if you didn't stop at the bucket you weren't giving it your all.

If you feel this coming on at the end of your interval or race, keep moving. Don't stop. The movement will help keep your heart pumping, the blood flowing, and flush out some of the lactic acid buildup. At the end of your workout it will also help your body adapt to a more static state. A proper cool down is always in order, good for the muscles, the body, and the soul. After that, you can hydrate and jump into the shower.

Ankle Sprains

Ankle sprains are more common in athletes participating in sports with side-to-side movement than that with straight-ahead motion. Court sports such as basketball, tennis, and racquetball all create a fair share of ankle sprains. Running on level ground does not often result in an ankle sprain, but cross-country running, trail running, and stepping in a pothole all could potentially lead to an ankle sprain. The most frequent ankle sprain is an inversion ankle sprain. This can injure the outer structures of the ankle.

The most common ankle injury resulting from an inversion is a partial tear of the anterior talo-fibular ligament. This ligament may also tear completely. The next most frequently injured ligament is the calcaneo-fibular ligament; the least injured is the posterior talo-fibular ligament. On occasion, the fibula itself may be fractured or the talar dome injured. As already mentioned, the other structures on the lateral side of the ankle should always be carefully examined to make sure they are not injured.

The grading of ankle sprains is officially done on an inadequate three-point scale. Grade 1 is a mild "stretch" of the ligaments, Grade 3 is a complete tear of the ligament, and Grade 2 is everything in between.

Treatment for Minor Sprains

It is impossible to guess how badly injured you are. If you have doubts, or if your ankle swells very rapidly, you should head for the emergency room. Immediate treatment should consist of RICE: Rest, Ice, Compression (gentle), and Elevation. The ice should be applied for about fifteen minutes at a time and then off for about the same. Avoid damaging your skin with the chemical bags you can place in your freezer. A bag of frozen corn or peas works just fine.

If the ankle does not respond quickly to this treatment, it is probably best to visit your sports physician for an evaluation and treatment. This way you'll avoid having your sprain be worse than a break.

For Grade 2 sprains an air cast is sometimes recommended to hold the ankle quiet as it heals and prevent further tearing or strain. On occasion, crutches are advised for a few days (or longer).

Starting to Exercise the Injury

The first exercise to try once the ankle is starting to feel better is dorsiflexion-plantarflexion, or just plain moving the ankle up and down. After more improvement, moving in small circles, painting the alphabet with your toes and other exercises can be done. Later still a theraband or other elastic band can be used to strengthen the muscles that help hold the ankle stable. Don't force your ankle to move in pain too soon, and avoiding weight bearing or walking in pain early in the course of an ankle sprain. There is no reason to start testing your ankle until it has had time to heal. Slow and easy gets more gain than rushing into painful exercises.

Heel Spurs and *Plantar Fasciitis*

A heel spur is a point of excess bone growth on the heel that usually extends forward towards the toes. Heel spurs are visible on X-ray.

The most common heel problems are actually caused by a painful tearing of the plantar fascia connecting the toes and the heel. (Plantar refers to the bottom of the foot and fascia is a type of dense fibrous connective tissue.) This may result in either a heel spur or *plantar fasciitis*.

If your foot flattens or becomes unstable during critical times in the walking or running cycle, the attachment of the plantar fascia into your heel bone may begin to stretch and pull away from the heel bone. This will result in pain and possibly swelling. The pain is especially noticeable when you push off with your toes while walking, since this movement stretches the already inflamed portion of the fascia.

Without treatment, the pain will usually spread around the heel. The pain is usually centered at a location just in front of the heel toward the arch. When the tearing occurs at the bone itself, the bone may attempt to heal itself by producing new bone. This results in the development of a heel spur. Without the spur the condition is called *plantar fasciitis*.

The pain of this condition may cause you to try to walk on your toes, or alter your running stride and gait, which will cause further damage and may cause a problem to develop in your healthy foot. Gait changes in running may also lead to ankle, knee, hip, or back pain.

Causes of Heel Spurs and *Plantar Fasciitis*

The most frequent cause of these injuries is an abnormal motion of the foot called excessive pronation. Normally, while walking or during long-distance running, your foot will strike the ground on the heel, then roll forward toward your toes and inward to the arch. Your arch should only dip slightly during this motion. If it lowers too much, you have what is known as excessive pronation. (For more details on pronation, see the section on biomechanics and gait in Chapter 13.)

The mechanical structure of your feet and the manner in which the different segments of your feet are linked together and joined with your legs has a major effect on their function and on the development of mechanically caused problems. Merely having "flat feet" won't take the spring out of your step, but having badly functioning feet with poor bone alignment will adversely affect the muscles, ligaments, and tendons and can create a variety of aches and pains. Excess pronation can cause the arch of your foot to stretch excessively with each step. It can also cause too much motion in segments of the foot that should be stable as you are walking or running. This "hypermobility" may cause other bones to shift and cause other mechanically induced problems.

Other factors that may contribute to *plantar fasciitis* and heel spurs include a sudden increase in daily activities, increase in weight (not usually a problem with runners), or a change of shoes. Dramatic increase in training intensity or duration may cause *plantar fasciitis*. Shoes that are too flexible in the middle of the arch or shoes that bend before the toe joints will cause an increase in tension in the plantar fascia. Make sure your shoes are not excessively worn.

Treatment of *Plantar Fasciitis*

As with most running-related injuries, an evaluation of changes in your training should be done. A decrease in workout intensity and duration is important. The most important part of self-treatment for this condition is being sure that your shoes offer motion control and are optimally controlling the forces that contribute to *plantar fasciitis* and heel spurs.

Check your running shoes to make sure that they are not excessively worn. They should bend only at the ball of the foot, where your toes attach to the foot. This is vital! Avoid any shoe that bends in the center of the arch or behind the ball of the foot. It offers insufficient support and will stress your plantar fascia. The human foot was not designed to bend here, and neither should a shoe be designed to do this.

Shoe Pushup Test

The "shoe pushup test" should be done to check where the shoe bends. Hold the heel of the shoe in one hand and then press up underneath the forefoot. The shoe should bend at the ball of the shoe, where the metatarsals would be. Next press under the part of the shoe where the metatarsal heads would be. The shoe should not bend under moderate pressure before this area. If it does you should change to a shoe that meets this criterion.

The treatment plan that seems to work best, with better than a 98 percent success rate, includes carefully following a program of physical therapy and strappings of the feet. The physical therapy modalities most frequently used include ultrasound (high frequency sound vibrations that create a deep heat and reduce inflammation) and galvanic (a carefully applied intermittent muscular stimulation to the heel and calf that helps reduce pain and relax muscle spasm which is a contributing factor to the pain). This treatment has been found most effective when given twice a week. The felt pads that will be strapped to your feet will compress after a few days and must be reapplied. While wearing them they should be kept dry, but may be removed the night before your next appointment.

Following control of the pain and inflammation associated with this injury, an orthotic should be used to stabilize your foot and prevent a recurrence. More than 98 percent of the time, heel spurs and *plantar fasciitis* can be controlled by this treatment, and surgery can be avoided. The orthotic prevents excess pronation and prevents lengthening of the plantar fascia and continued tearing of the fascia. Usually a slight heel lift and a firm shank in the shoe will also help to reduce the severity of this problem.

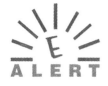

It is important to be aware of how your foot feels over this time period. If your foot is still uncomfortable without the strapping but was more comfortable while wearing it, that is an indication that the treatment should help. Remember, what took many months or years to develop cannot be eliminated in just a few days.

Neuroma Pain

Neuroma pain is classically described as a burning pain in the forefoot. It can also be felt as an aching or shooting pain in the forefoot. Patients with this problem frequently say they feel like they want to take off their shoes and rub their foot. It may occur in the middle of a run or at the end of a long run. If your shoes are quite tight it may occur very early in the run.

Causes of Neuroma Pain

The source of this pain is an enlargement of the sheath of an intermetatarsal nerve in the foot. This usually occurs in the third intermetatarsal space, the space between the third and fourth toes and metatarsals. It occurs here because this is the area in which the intermetatarsal nerve is thickest because it is made up of the joining of several different nerves.

Pronation of the foot can cause the metatarsal heads to rotate slightly and pinch the nerve that runs between the metatarsal heads. This chronic pinching can make the nerve sheath enlarge. As it enlarges, it becomes more squeezed and increasingly troublesome.

Treating Neuroma

Treatment of this condition is mostly practical and has a lot to do with your shoes. It includes wearing shoes with a wide toe box, not lacing the forefoot part of your shoe too tight, and making sure your feet are in supportive shoes but not being squeezed. If this doesn't relieve the pain, work with a doctor to decide on these treatments: orthotics, an injection of steroids, or surgical removal of the neuroma, preferably in that order.

Shin Splints

In the past, the term shin splint was medically used to encompass almost all problems occurring in the lower leg. These problems included both bone and soft tissue problems and those that overlapped. They were jumbled into several categories that poorly represented reality. The previous categories in use were anterior, posterior, medial, and lateral. Now, doctors use the terms medial tibial stress syndrome, compartment syndrome, and stress fracture to describe injuries of the lower leg.

Most athletes have used the term shin splint to refer to pain occurring either in the anterior or the medial portion of the leg. This correlates well with the type of problems that are most often clinically seen and will be discussed here. Problems that occur in the lateral aspect of the leg are usually either fibular stress fractures or peroneal tendon injuries following an inversion injury of the ankle. Posterior leg pains are frequently injuries to the posterior muscle group at the myotendinous junction of the calf muscles and Achilles tendon or early Achilles tendonitis.

Medial Shin Splints

The outmoded term *medial shin splints* has been replaced by the term *medial tibial stress syndrome* (MTSS). Either term suffices to describe pain at the medial aspect of the leg, adjacent to the medial tibia. Tenderness is usually found between three and twelve centimeters above the tip of the medial malleolus at the posterio-medial aspect of the tibia.

When the tibia is palpated (touched), the tenderness is not directly medial but is just behind the most medial portion of the tibia, in the mass of soft tissue that is there and at the bone itself. Periostitis sometimes occurs in this location. The sore, inflamed structures usually include the medial muscles and tendons here. Most frequently involved is the posterior tibial tendon and muscle, but the *flexor digitorum longus* and *flexor hallucis longus* may also be involved.

Stress fractures can also occur in this area. The definitive test for stress fracture is a bone scan, but false negatives can occur and it is possible that a false positive might occur also, because of the soft tissue and periosteal involvement in this injury. Clinically, physical examination can be used to differentiate between medial shin splints and a stress fracture. With medial shin splints, the tenderness extends along a considerable vertical distance of the tibia. When a stress fracture is present, tenderness is usually noted that extends horizontally across the front of the tibia.

Risk Factors

The first risk factor is overtraining. Evaluate your schedule to determine what training errors you may have made. Mechanically, pronation is most likely to be the culprit. When the foot pronates, the medial structures of the leg are stretched and put under stress, and this increases the likelihood that they will become injured. Running on a cambered surface, such as the side of a crowned road, can put the upper leg at risk to develop this problem, because the foot of the upper leg is functioning in a pronated position.

Treating MTSS

Decrease training immediately. Do not run if pain occurs during or following your run. Non-weight bearing exercise may be necessary. Swimming, biking, and pool running can all be used to maintain fitness. While running on soft surfaces has been recommended for this problem, that is not likely to help a pure MTSS. The foot is more likely to pronate excessively on mushy grass or sand. Packed dirt is ideal, and avoidance of concrete is also helpful.

In many cases, shoes that are rated high for control of pronation may be helpful. Gentle posterior stretching exercises may help, but control of pronation is more directly related to the cause of this syndrome. Ice applications following running may offer some relief, but are not curative. If symptoms persist it is important to seek professional medical attention.

In-office medical care will repeat some of the procedures that you have done. A thorough evaluation of your training schedule, racing schedule, and shoes will be followed by a biomechanical evaluation. Anti-inflammatory medication can be prescribed. The use of physical therapy modalities such as electrical stimulation (HVGS) and ultrasound can also be helpful to treat this problem, as can taping the foot to limit pronation and decrease the stress on the medial structures of the leg. Pronation, which is a major contributing factor to this syndrome, in the long run, may be approached with improved shoes and over-the-counter or custom orthotics.

Anterior Shin Splints

The medical term anterior shin splints has been replaced in the past three years. Now the symptoms that occur in the anterior lateral tibial region are assumed to be either stress fractures or a form of compartment syndrome. In understanding the anterior shin splint, it is important to differentiate shin splint from a stress fracture.

Most injuries that fit the term "anterior shin splint" are soft tissue injuries at the muscular origin and bony or periosteal interface of the bone and muscle origin. These usually have a longer more vertically oriented area of symptoms and tenderness.

The involved section of the upper tibia is usually five to eight centimeters long and about one to two centimeters wide. Most injuries that clinically seem to be stress fractures have what is called a region of pinpoint tenderness and extend in a horizontal direction. The tenderness is pinpoint in respect to the fact that a discrete line of tenderness exists, not a pinpoint shape. This line in many stress fractures of the tibia extends horizontally, but might take a tangential course through the tibia. With those that are horizontal there would be no tenderness found one or two centimeters above or below this discrete line of tenderness.

The non-stress fracture injury to this area may be due to micro-tears of the muscle either at the origin or in the fibers themselves. This may occur because of repetitive traction or pulling of the anterior tibial muscles at their site of origin. Repetitive loading with excessive stress, such as that caused by running on concrete, may also play a role in injury to this area. This may result in micro-trauma to the bone structure itself.

Anterior Compartment Syndrome

One should be aware that a compartment syndrome can occur here. This is usually chronic and repetitive and in some respects different from the acute compartment syndrome seen after serious muscle injuries. It is vital to seek evaluation and treatment, if this is suspected. It is caused by the muscles swelling within a closed compartment with a resultant increase in pressure in the compartment. The blood supply can be compromised and muscle injury and pain may occur. The symptoms include leg pain, unusual nerve sensations (paresthesia), and, later, muscle weakness. Definitive evaluation is done by measuring the pressure in the compartment. Surgical decompression of the compartment may be required to relieve the pain.

Runners at Risk for Anterior Shin Splints

The usual runners at risk for anterior shin splints are beginning runners. These runners have not acclimated to the stresses of running yet. They also may not have been doing an adequate amount of stretching. Poor choice of shoes and surface (i.e. concrete) can also play a role. Overtraining, of course, can be one of the factors in problems here as in most other running injuries.

The usual mechanical factors seen are an imbalance between the posterior and anterior muscle groups. The posterior muscles may be both too tight and too strong. The effect of too tight posterior musculature has ramifications for the gait cycle at two points.

The first time in which too tight posterior muscles have an impact on the anterior muscles is just before and after foot contact (heel for the distance runner). At this time the anterior muscles are acting as decelerators. If the posterior muscles are too tight they will force the anterior muscles to work longer and harder in this deceleration.

The second point in the gait cycle where the anterior muscles may work too hard is when the foot leaves the ground, at toe off. The anterior muscles should be lifting up, or dorsiflexing, the foot at this time, so that the toes will clear the ground as the leg is brought forward. If the posterior muscles are too tight, the anterior muscles again will be working harder than they should be. Logically, downhill running will also have an adverse effect on the anterior muscles.

Repetitive impact on hard surfaces is another frequently associated factor. Excessive pronation may be a minor factor, but it is a much greater factor in the medial tibial stress syndrome (medial shin splints).

Self-Care

Decrease training immediately. Do not run if pain occurs during or following your run. Non-weight bearing exercise may be necessary. The goal will be to find the distance that can be run, if any, that does not produce symptoms—not to find what your real limit is. Swimming, biking, and pool running can all be used to maintain fitness. Review your stretching and think about what good habits can keep you out of the doctor's office.

The posterior muscles should be gently stretched (see both Chapter 7 and the stretching tips in Chapter 13). It's recommended that you do gentle stretching of the calf muscles and the hamstrings.

Shoes with too many miles on them should be replaced. Shock absorption should be a factor in selecting shoes in the individual with anterior shin splints. Downhill running can aggravate this problem and should be avoided. Too long a stride can also delay healing. Most of all, *do not run on concrete*. After exercise, apply an icepack to lessen symptoms.

Office Medical Care of Anterior Shin Splints

In-office medical care will repeat some of the procedures that you have done. A thorough evaluation of your training schedule, racing schedule, and shoes will be followed by a biomechanical evaluation. A bone scan can be used, if necessary, to evaluate for the possibility of stress fracture. A wick catheter test can be used, if necessary, to measure post exercise compartment pressure, if a compartment syndrome is suspected.

Anti-inflammatory medication can be prescribed. The use of physical therapy modalities can also be helpful. I use electrical stimulation

(HVGS) to treat this problem. Sometimes a heel lift is used to reduce the pulling effect of tight posterior muscles. While this does increase the distance the foot must be dorsiflexed, the duration of action and the effective strength of the posterior muscles is decreased. Orthotics may also be considered when biomechanical abnormalities exist and problems persist.

Anterior Ankle Pain

The tendons in front of your ankle can sometimes get irritated when the tongue continues up around the front of the ankle and is compressed by the laces. This can also impinge upon the nerves in this area with the result being an occasional numbness, but most often pain. Of course other things can cause pain in this area, such as injuries to the ligaments or bones. Try skipping the top lace completely rather than just lacing it looser. You can than lace your shoe securely without irritation. Odds are this should help a lot. If this simple solution doesn't work, get it checked by a sports medicine practitioner.

Selecting a Sports Physician

It is important to choose a doctor who has had experience in treating athletes. The telephone directory is a poor guide to this. Try speaking to other runners for a recommendation. You may contact a local running club or a reputable running shoe store for their suggestions. It is vital that you choose someone with both experience and a good reputation among runners.

A question that is often asked and subject to much debate is whether your doctor should be a runner. This is not a good question. This makes as much sense as seeking an oncologist to evaluate and treat your cancer based on his own personal history of cancer. While the doctor being an athlete may add to his understanding of both the psyche and the physical conditions that lead to injury, it is not a prerequisite to being capable of appropriately treating your problem. The recommendations of knowledgeable people are the most valuable resource for finding a capable sports medicine physician.

Board Certification

In spite of the popular press suggesting that your sports physician be board certified in sports medicine, there are no organizations that currently render a board certified status to any physician or podiatric physician. Fellowship status may be achieved, however, by qualification and testing by the American College of Sports Medicine and the American Academy of Podiatric Sports Medicine.

A Certificate of Added Qualifications in Sports Medicine may also be granted if one meets multiple criteria and successfully passes a certifying examination. This exam is given and the certification granted through a joint venture by the American Board of Family Practice, American Board of Pediatrics, American Board of Internal Medicine, and American Board of Emergency Medicine.

Other medical organizations of sports medicine include the American Orthopedic Society of Sports Medicine and the American Medical Society of Sports Medicine. Organizations that may help you find a capable sports medicine practitioner are the American Running and Fitness Association, the American Academy of Podiatric Sports Medicine, and the American College of Sports Medicine.

CHAPTER 15
All About Nutrition

Nutrition is one of the most important considerations runners face, especially as they begin to build toward longer runs and marathons. Eating right is a major contributor to your overall comfort level and an enhanced performance. The information in this chapter will keep you up to date with current medical thinking regarding sports nutrition.

A Nutritious Mindset

What to eat, when to eat, even how to eat—all of this we learn from our parents and peers. Really, it's not until we're teenagers that we have much of a choice about what we eat. And then, of course, it becomes fun to eat all the "bad" stuff—fast food, high-fat snacks, pizza with extra, extra cheese. It becomes easy and gratifying to include these foods as part of our regular meals. And then, of course, they become habits. Habits that lead to weight gain, lethargy, and even addiction. Yikes!

When a Diet Isn't a Diet

A diet is actually what makes up the foods you live on day after day. It doesn't matter whether you eat poorly or well; your diet is the foods you consume. Period. In the United States, though, diet has come to mean what we're restricted to eat in order to lose weight. Because most of us have been on diets, and certainly we're all exposed to the diet culture, it's hard not to think of any kind of diet as one that leads to tough choices, over-conscientious eating, and ultimately, frustration.

One of the things you have to mentally overcome is thinking of your diet as a faddish weight-loss plan. Instead, think of your diet as the fuel that feeds your machine (your body). Do you want to keep filling up your tank with crud that ultimately leads to break-downs, or do you want to put in the kind of fuel that keeps things running at their very best and that guarantees performance? If you're reading this book and are serious about your fitness and training, you undoubtedly chose the latter.

Nutrition Know-How

To get the most out of the fuel you put into your body, you have to understand what makes up the fuel. What is in the fuel that provides energy? What is in the fuel that is wasteful or harmful? What is the right balance of nutrients that will help you feel your best? What nutritionists, doctors, and scientists have found to be optimal is a meal that breaks out thusly: 55 to 60 percent of total calories from carbohydrates, 25 percent of total calories from fat, and 15 percent of total calories from protein. These are three of the six essential nutrients your body needs. The others are water, vitamins, and minerals. All will be discussed in this chapter.

The chemical processes in your body that break down and utilize nutrients food are called your metabolism. Everyone's metabolism is different, which is why some people can seemingly eat anything and never gain weight, while others need to be constantly thinking about the amount they eat.

Carbohydrates

A really simplified way to think of carbohydrates is by this rhyme: Carbohydrates come from the ground, proteins run around. This means carbohydrates are typically grains, fruits, and vegetables (and proteins are typically meats). In reality, it's more complicated than that. Carbohydrates are actually the sugars, starches, and cellulose the body needs for energy. They come in two forms: complex carbohydrates and simple carbohydrates.

Complex Carbohydrates

Complex carbohydrates are what are most commonly referred to as "carbs." Chemically more complex than simple carbohydrates, they also take longer to break down and enter the bloodstream. They are higher in fiber and lower in fat and calories than simple carbohydrates, and they last longer to give the body energy over longer periods of time. The body stores complex carbohydrates in the liver and muscles as glycogen.

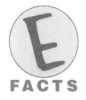

Complex carbohydrates are found in vegetables, beans, grain, and pasta. Some high-quality complex carbohydrates are brown rice, whole grains, broccoli, dried peas, beans and lentils, corn, bananas and other fresh and dried fruits, pumpkin, sweet potatoes, and of course, pasta.

Simple Carbohydrates

Simple carbohydrates are the ones that give you instant energy. Their molecular structure is simpler than their complex counterparts, so their energy gets into your system quite rapidly. They also have a shorter lifespan and are typically lower in fiber and higher in calories. Common simple carbohydrates are found in processed sugar and other processed foods, and some fruits. Examples include white bread, potato chips, fried rice, sweetened cereals, and so on.

Fats

If there's a nutrient with a bad rap, it's fat. But notice, fat should make up a slightly greater percentage of your daily food than protein! That's because fat supplies essential fatty acids, which supply energy for aerobic activities like walking and climbing stairs. Stored fat insulates vital organs and transports fat-soluble vitamins (A, D, E, and K). Fat can be your friend! Like carbohydrates, there are also two kinds of fat: saturated and unsaturated.

Saturated Fats

Saturated fats are the bad kind—those that block your arteries and don't make much of a contribution to your overall health. You still need some of them, but not much; restrict them to about 10 percent of your total calories (less than one-third of your total fat intake). You'll find saturated fats in whole dairy products such as butter, cheese and ice cream; coconut, cottonseed, and palm kernel oils; and in beef, pork, ham, and sausage.

Unsaturated Fats

Unsaturated fats come in two varieties: monounsaturated and polyunsaturated. Monounsaturated fats are those in olive and canola oils, whereas corn, safflower, soybean, and sunflower oils all contain polyunsaturated fats.

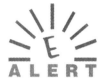

Otherwise known as hydrogenated vegetable oils, the body recognizes and uses trans-fatty acids (TFAs) as saturated fats. Hydrogenation is the process of adding hydrogen to polyunsaturated fats to give foods a longer shelf life and added flavor. They're found in cookies, crackers, and fried foods.

Protein

Considered the building block for all tissues and cells, protein's primary function is to build and repair red blood cells, muscle, hair, and cells for body tissues. Protein is a secondary energy provider (to carbohydrates). It's in meat, fish, dairy products like cheese, milk, and yogurt, and in the edible parts of leguminous plants like beans, peas, and lentils.

Water

You could survive for many days without food, but without water you could die quite rapidly. The human body is 60–70 percent water, and needs to be replenished constantly. It is responsible for transporting nutrients, gases, and waste products, and for regulating your body's temperature. Water is not only vitally necessary for good health, it has side benefits of being able to cool or heat your body as well as moisturize and soothe your insides (and skin!). It can also help you feel full and curb your appetite.

Drinking Enough Water

It's difficult to drink too much water in the course of a day—you can have as much as you want! The recommended amount for adults is sixty-four ounces, or eight eight-ounce servings. The truth is, most people don't drink enough water. They're more accustomed to drinking soda, juice, coffee, tea, or alcohol. How often have you heard that you'll feel better by just getting in your sixty-four ounces of water every day? Well, it's true.

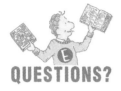

What's the best way to get the water you need?
Try this:

With breakfast: Eight ounces
Between 8:00 A.M. and 12:00 P.M.: Twenty-four ounces
With lunch: Eight ounces
Between 1:30 and 6:30: Sixteen ounces
With dinner: Eight ounces

If you have another sixteen ounces between dinner and when you go to bed, you'll even exceed your daily minimum requirement. Way to go!

Hydrating Versus Dehydrating Fluids

You could argue that since many beverages are made with water they should be counted towards your daily sixty-four ounces. You'd be correct with some of them, incorrect with others. Hydrating beverages, which all contribute to the improved functioning of your body, include (besides water) sports drinks that replace electrolytes, fruit juices (the less sugar, the better), soy or rice beverages (great whole milk replacements), herbal teas, and milk.

It doesn't help to cheat here, though. Milk may be hydrating, for example, but it's not a good idea to drink much more than sixteen ounces of it a day, particularly if it's whole milk. And while juices do contain fruit, most of the readily available juices have sugar as their main ingredient (a simple carb that'll lift you up and drop you down).

Dehydrating fluids contain water, but they also rob your body of water. These are caffeinated and alcoholic beverages. To minimize their effect, drink water in a 1:1 ratio with them.

Vitamins and Minerals

There's a vitamin for practically every letter in the alphabet, sometimes even a few with the same letter. This can get very confusing! Why are there so many vitamins? Because vitamins perform a lot of functions in the body. For example, vitamin A is a moisturizer for your skin and mucous membranes and also aids vision. Meanwhile, vitamin C is responsible for intracellular maintenance of bone, capillaries, and teeth, and vitamin E protects polyunsaturated fats and prevents cell membrane damage.

Simplify your thinking about vitamins by remembering that the best way to get essential vitamins is through your food. So if you're eating right (according to your size, stress, and exercise-level requirements), chances are you're getting most of the vitamins you need. With demanding lifestyles and reliance on more and more packaged and processed foods, however, vitamin supplements can be helpful.

Like vitamins, minerals are necessary to aid and induce a number of vital bodily functions. For instance, calcium aids bones, teeth, blood clotting, and nerve and muscle function. Magnesium aids bone growth and nerve, muscle, and enzyme function, while phosphorous aids bone, teeth, and energy transfer.

Unfortunately, having a healthy diet is not as easy as taking a lot of supplements. In fact, crashing on any minerals or vitamins can be dangerous, because it can disrupt your body's balance in any of these areas. All foods work together to provide your body with the six essential nutrients it needs: carbohydrates, fats, proteins, water, vitamins, and minerals.

Fiber and Cholesterol

There are a couple of other things that contribute nutritionally to your overall health that aren't included in the Big Six. These are fiber and cholesterol.

Fiber is an essential aid in healthy digestion because it cannot be digested. It is the "roughage" that passes through our system, attracting and absorbing water, digested food, and cholesterol. The source of fiber is the plant cell walls, which are broken down considerably during the processing of food. Consequently, there is less and less natural fiber in our daily diet. There are two types of fiber, soluble and insoluble, and the recommended amount is about thirty grams (combined).

Insoluble fiber attracts water and digested food; soluble fiber goes the extra mile and gets cholesterol. Fiber-rich foods include whole grains, fruits, and vegetables. Drinking lots of water also helps fiber do its job.

Like discussions about fat, those about cholesterol are usually negative. Excess cholesterol sticks to the walls of your arteries, causing blockage. The source of cholesterol is animal-based food products: meat, fish, poultry, eggs, and dairy products.

However, cholesterol is important to our health. It aids in the synthesis of adrenal (kidney) and sex hormones, and vitamin D and bile. Cholesterol is naturally produced in the liver. The Food and Drug Administration recommends consuming less than 300 milligrams per day of cholesterol.

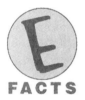

FACTS

Do you like cheeseburgers, omelets, and ice cream? Here's how the cholesterol stacks up in them:

1 ground beef patty (medium-sized): 74 mg
1 cup shredded cheddar cheese: 119 mg
1 hardboiled or poached egg: 212 mg (all from the yolk)
1 cup ice cream: up to 290 mg

Eating Right for Running

Now it's time to learn how to turn nutrition knowledge into sound food choices that will enable you to perform at an optimal level while feeling better overall. Remember, it's not just about losing weight, it's about properly fueling the daily activities you want to undertake so that you can fully participate in and enjoy them.

It Starts in the Brain

How do you know when you're hungry? Does your stomach grumble? Perhaps. Do you feel distracted, as if you're waiting for something to happen? Probably. Have you been so hungry sometimes that you feel like you could eat almost anything? So hungry that you get impatient waiting or looking for something to eat? When you have any of these feelings, it means your brain is glucose-deprived.

When your brain isn't getting the fuel it needs, besides making you feel ravenous, it can also make you feel shaky, irritable, indecisive, sluggish, and headachy. A part of your subconscious brain takes over and sends out survival signals to eat. This typically leads to poor nutritional choices, whether it's because you wolf down some nutrient-poor snacks or junk food, or because you eat too much too quickly.

Satisfying Your Mind and Your Body

To supply your body with the energy it needs you need to be aware of three things:

1. The types of food and beverages you are consuming
2. The amounts you are eating or drinking
3. The timing, or when you are eating and drinking

What you need is a basic plan about how to eat so that these three requirements are met and your body has what it needs to maximize energy and achieve metabolic maintenance. This is particularly important as a runner, because, like a car heading out on a long trip, you need all your fluids topped to operate in your best form.

Pace and Calories

It has been estimated that between 100–120 calories are burned per mile. This appears to be fairly constant and independent of running speed. Although there is a slight increase of rate of calorie burning with an increase in speed, it is considered negligible. One of the obvious advantages of running, when it comes to burning calories, is the shorter time it takes to burn the same number of calories, when compared to walking bicycling, swimming, and most other aerobic exercises. Many physiologists also feel that the metabolic rate remains higher for several hours after exercise. Runners often notice a decrease in appetite after a good run. On the other hand, with all this increase in burning of calories, more food can safely be enjoyed!

How to Eat

Studies have shown that the most effective way to feed your body is by eating breakfast, snacking, eating two to three hours before going to sleep, and manipulating your fat-cell storage.

Eating Breakfast

After even a mere four to five hours of sleep, when you awake in the morning your body is coming out of a fasting period. The fuel tank is on low or empty. Even if you don't feel hungry in the morning, it's important to "break the fast" and replenish the nutrients. This prevents your brain from sending out hunger-alert signals later in the morning and stabilizes your energy needs for later in the day. Psychologically, having something to eat in the morning can also prevent you from feeling like you can overindulge later to make up for the skipped meal.

Snacking

If you were raised to refrain from snacking because it ruined your appetite for your main meals, this will be a tough habit to form. If you are a snacker already, but you feel you are overweight, you may want to examine the types of snacks you're eating and when you're eating them. Let's be clear: A snack is a small amount of food eaten between meals whose purpose is to prevent blood sugar levels from dropping too low. The best snacks are those made up of complex carbohydrates that are low in fat and high in fiber, such as fruit, whole grains, and some vegetables.

Snacking, also referred to as "grazing," is actually the preferred way to eat. Rather than consuming three large meals (breakfast, lunch, and dinner), grazing means spreading your total caloric intake throughout the day, eating smaller yet satisfying portions of food every three or so hours.

Eating Well Before Going to Sleep

After you eat, your body gets busy processing its food. This is called digestion. The body also has a long "to-do" list for the time that you're asleep. If the body needs to digest and tackle its to-do list at the same time (meaning you've eaten just before going to sleep), it's not going to be able to do its best work. It's like your boss giving you an extra assignment just as you're about to quit for the day. Make every effort to eat a small, healthy snack two to three hours before you go to sleep if you want your body to process the food to the best of its ability.

Eating for the Early Morning Runner

For many people, the best time to run is when they first get up in the morning, before the commitments of family and work. With all this discussion about how important it is to break the night's fast and have enough fuel for the day, are runners who work out before breakfast ultimately causing their bodies to store fat?

In general, getting a run in before breakfast is fine so long as you aren't skipping breakfast altogether. Optimally, you want to ingest some form of complex carbohydrate and fluid before you set off. A big glass of orange juice (with pulp) along with a glass of water will help. After your run and five to ten minutes of stretching, when you've cooled off, have a bagel, whole grain bread or cereal, some fruit, and lots of water for breakfast. Don't try Rocky's early-morning fix of five raw eggs. It doesn't taste good and it's not good for you!

Getting into Eating

Now that you have an understanding of nutrition and know that you need to graze at intervals throughout the day, it's time to get to the heart of the matter: What to eat and in what quantities.

Using the premise that food is energy, how much energy you expend determines how much food you should eat. This is called your daily caloric need, and it's something that can change even daily depending on what comes up in your life (longer runs = greater energy needs; more stress = greater energy needs; more sedentary lifestyle = fewer energy needs, etc.).

The first thing you need to do is create an objective nutritional analysis for yourself to see where you are with your eating habits. There are whole fields of study devoted to this, and this book can't answer all your questions. You can read other books on the subject or you can ask your doctor to refer you to a specialist. What this book will do is lay the groundwork for you.

Your Eating Habits

Do you even know how much and when you eat during a typical day? Most people don't. The best way to learn is to keep a food journal for at least a week. Using a notebook, your Palm Pilot, your running log, or a calendar—something you can keep a record in—begin to write down everything you eat and when you eat it. Don't cheat! You must even list the breath mints you chew in between meetings. If you can, it's helpful to note where you were eating, too. At your desk while you finished a report? In the cafeteria? In front of the TV?

After a week, which includes a weekend, you'll have a good idea of the what, when, and where of your eating habits. Even from the brief discussion in this book, you should be able to see where you're making your nutritional "no-no"s based on your food diary. How often did you skip breakfast? How often did you eat high-fat foods like junk food, desserts, or fried food? What are your snacking habits? How many fruits and vegetables do you eat in a typical week?

Fat Cell Storage

Irregular eating causes your brain to protect your fat cells, because those are what hold energy. If you have a track record of skipping meals and eating erratically, you've trained your body to store fat, which is why it might be more difficult for you to lose weight. Eating regularly and healthfully means the brain doesn't have to worry about energy sources, which means your fat cells won't be stored up—it'll be used as it should be.

Where You Are Versus Where You Need to Be

To make intelligent food choices easier, the U.S. government has dietary guidelines recommended by the American Dietetic Association, American Cancer Society, American College of Sports Medicine, American Heart Association, and the surgeon general. The recommendations are that your intake at every meal should be made up of 55 to 60 percent carbohydrates, 20 to 30 percent fats (no more than 10 percent from saturated fat), and 10 to 15 percent proteins. This is the combination that works best to fuel all your systems and provide balance in your diet.

Looking at food as percentages makes meal planning easier. Endurance athletes often push their carbohydrate intake to 65 percent while offsetting this by reducing their total fat calories. If you were to apply this to your plate at mealtime, you'd see that the section for carbs is the largest, protein next, and fat smallest (because even though the percentage recommendation is higher, it has twice the caloric value as carbs).

ESSENTIALS Using these recommendations, look back at your food log for the week and chart your main meals by whether they were largely composed of carbs, protein, or fat. Surprised? Apply these recommendations at restaurants and while grocery shopping. Are meats and ice cream taking up more room than fresh vegetables, whole grains, and fresh fruit?

Eating Smart at Restaurants

Don't forget to eat smart when dining out. Even many of the fast-food restaurants out there have some healthy options on their menus. You can even eat healthy in fine restaurants by asking for salad dressing, butter, and sour cream on the side so that you can control the portions of these high-fat condiments. Ask for chicken or fish entrées to be broiled rather than fried. When perusing restaurant menus that offer lots of high-fat food options, keeping in mind that you are an athlete in search of performance fuel will bolster your willpower to make sound nutritional choices.

As a runner, this information is especially valuable. To eat right for running, you need the nutrients that will best fuel your energy. These are carbohydrates. But proteins are essential for aiding in the utilization of energy, and fat is essential for overall good health. Please use these chapters as your introduction to nutrition and healthy eating. There are many other sources of information to study and follow. And if you're not feeling well for any reason, consult with your physician.

The Food Guide Pyramid

The U.S. Department of Agriculture created the Food Guide Pyramid to help simplify healthy eating. It breaks out food by the number of recommended servings that should be eaten daily (see **FIGURE 15-1**). A serving is considered approximately a half-cup of the food source (pasta and rice, for example), or a couple of slices of bread, a whole fruit such as an apple, a couple of large carrots, an eight-ounce yogurt, a half-pound serving of fish or meat, etc.

ALERT

At the top of the food guide pyramid, in the smallest part, is the recommendation for fats, oils, and sweets. All the other groups have serving amounts next to them. Not this one. They are to be eaten "sparingly." You know what that means: keep the Snickers bars and sodas to a minimum.

THE USDA FOOD GUIDE PYRAMID

Fats, oils, and sweets
USE SPARINGLY ────────────►

Key
- Fat (naturally occurring and added)
- ▼ Sugars (added)

These symbols show fat, oils, and added sugars in foods.

Milk, yogurt, and cheese group
2–3 SERVINGS ───────►

Meat, poultry, fish, dry beans, eggs, and nuts group
◄─────────── **2–3 SERVINGS**

Vegetable group
3–5 SERVINGS ───────►

Fruit group
◄─────────── **2–4 SERVINGS**

Bread, cereal, rice, and pasta group
◄─────────── **6–11 SERVINGS**

The USDA Food Guide Pyramid helps guide you toward the types and numbers of food servings. United States Department of Agriculture and Health and Human Services: The food guide pyramid.

COMMON SOURCES OF CARBOHYDRATE, PROTEIN, AND FAT

Macronutrient	Food sources
Carbohydrates	
Starches	Pasta, rice, grains, breads, cereals, potatoes, dried beans, and peas
Sugars	Fruits, candy, cookies, cakes, jelly, sugar, honey, syrup, molasses, soda pop
Protein	Meats, fish, poultry, eggs, milk, yogurt, cheese, nuts, dried beans
Fat	
Saturated	Animal fats, butter, cheese, whole milk, mayonnaise, egg yolks, ice cream, chocolate, lard, hydrogenated oils, coconut and palm oils
Polyunsaturated	Some margarines, nuts, and oils (i.e., corn, safflower, soybean, cottonseed, sesame, and sunflower oils)
Monounsaturated	Olive, canola, and peanut oils

From "The Food Guide Pyramid" by U.S. Department of Agriculture, Human Nutrition Information Service, 1992, Leaflet No. 572, U.S. Government Printing Office, Washington, D.C.

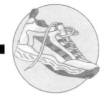

CHAPTER 16

Are You Ready for the Marathon?

The marathon is one of the most grueling events in all of sports. It requires long months of painstaking training and planning. Finishing one is one of the most rewarding experiences any runner can possibly imagine. It takes dedication, resolve, and persistence. It is also something that should only be attempted by a runner who has some miles under his or her belt. It is not something to be taken lightly.

Deciding If You're Ready for the Marathon

You should not be attempting a marathon unless you have been running at least one year and are comfortably running twenty-five miles a week or more. If you find that running twenty-five miles per week is difficult for you to accomplish for any number of reasons (aches and pains, time constraints, etc.), you are not yet ready to begin training for this event.

In this chapter you'll learn about the history of the marathon, which is rich with legend and excitement. You'll also get training schedules, complete with advice on precautions you should take, experimentation you might want to do, along with psychological strategies that you can employ before, during, and after the marathon.

The History of the Marathon

There is probably no sporting event in the world that has more history tied to it than the marathon. It is legend. And as with all legends, the story has been twisted and retold many times. The following story of where the marathon began and how it got its name is the best version that can be found, and is probably the most correct.

Greece and the Persian Empire

The marathon was named for the battle of Marathon, a large plain in Greece located approximately twenty-five miles from Athens. Back in 490 B.C., King Xerxes was trying to find a way toward Europe over land. He was the king of the Persian Empire, which stretched from Asia through Egypt and into the Mediterranean via the Red Sea.

The Greek and Persian wars took place in the fifth century B.C. In their quest for expansion, the Persians had taken several of the smaller city-states, most notably Iona. They had conquered the city and then later brutally crushed an uprising against Persian control. To gain the control of the passage by land to the rest of Europe, Greece had to be dominated.

Persia's army was at this time in history seemingly invincible, as it had laid waste to many armies under the direction of their famous general,

Darius. For Persia, Greece was a stumbling block. On the seas Persia could not defeat Greece, which at that time was a group of loosely bound together city-states that practiced a new form of governance called democracy.

To conquer Greece, Persia needed to defeat the two main city-states, Sparta and Athens. Athens was the largest polis (city-state), the center of democracy and culture. Sparta was a military state, very rigid and conservative, with a king and a ruling class. Sparta and Athens had fought each other often, but they easily agreed to join together to fend off the onslaught of the Persian threat.

As the Athenians drew close to the field to confirm the enormity of the Persian presence, a runner was dispatched to Sparta, 150 miles away, to warn them of the invasion and to ask for their aid. The messenger's name was Philippides.

The Spartans, after being notified of the Persian landing, agreed to send troops to aid the Atheneans, but would not leave Sparta until the full moon, which was the established law. As the Athenians were trying to hold out for the Spartans, the Persians decided to force their hand. They began dividing their soldiers, with the plan of attacking the city while the army was held at bay in Marathon. It's estimated that the Athenians were outnumbered approximately four to one.

With their backs against the wall, the Athenians hatched a bold plan. They launched a massive assault that seemed suicidal. They presented their army as a broad front, but in fact had many of their men either positioned or moved to the flanks the nearer they came to the approaching Persians. The Persians were actually astonished by what they considered a sad and foolhardy attempt to rush them.

In response, they formed an even line across, and loaded up the middle, hoping to break the Athenian center. The Athenians outflanked the Persians, confusion reigned as the Persians were suddenly surrounded, and the slaughter was on. By most accounts 6,000 to 7,000 Persians lay dead on the field of battle, next to less than 200 Athenians.

However, the battle was not yet over. Another Persian force was sent to take the city after the battle. By that time the Spartans had arrived to assist in battle, and the Spartans and the Athenians turned back the

Persians yet again. With this victory, the tide of world history had been irrevocably changed. The Persian-Greek wars did not stop, but the myth of Persian invincibility was forever shattered.

Philippides, the Runner

This is where the story goes a little awry. The "legend" has it that Philippides ran from Marathon to Athens and uttered, "Victory!" or "Rejoice, we conquer!" reporting on the battle, then died, spent and exhausted. This account survived for centuries. But the truth is that the stories of Philippides, hardly mentioned in the accounts written just after the battle, became popular 600 years after the fact.

Was it really Philippides who ran the 150 miles in two days? Perhaps not, but someone definitely did, and that is a feat enough in itself. In actuality, it's unlikely the same runner would have been sent back to Marathon, then to Athens from Marathon, even though runners were a common way to communicate vital information.

The Marathon at the Olympics

The first Olympic games were held sometime between 1200 B.C. and 800 B.C. The years between 776 B.C. and A.D. 394 were the golden age of Greek athletics, where the Olympic prize was the ultimate goal for thousands of talented amateurs and professionals. So important were the games that wars between the city-states were suspended so that the games could take place.

Because of the games' religious significance to the Greek people, the Roman Emperor Theodosious banned the Olympics in A.D. 394, as they were a slight to Christian hegemony.

There were several unsuccessful attempts to revive the Olympics in the 1800s by a wealthy Greek businessman named Evangelios Zappas. Attempts in 1859, 1870, 1875, and 1889 all failed to provide the kind of pageantry and high-caliber competition deserving of Olympics. But Pierre de Coubertain, a French baron, in an attempt to bridge two of his favorite causes—health through athleticism and international cooperation in Europe—dreamed up an international contest of athletics. He introduced many of the themes into the Olympics that we associate with them today. At a conference to establish the Olympics, another Frenchman proposed a race to commemorate Phillipides run from Marathon, and an incredible distance run was established as the final event of the games.

The First Olympic Games

In 1896, the first modern Olympic Games were held in Athens. On the final day of the meet, the Greeks had not yet won a gold medal. The big race loomed as their last chance. The course began at the Marathon Bridge and went to the Olympic Stadium, a distance of 40,000 meters, or 24.85 miles. In an almost preordained salute to the victory in Marathon so many centuries before, a Greek runner, Spiridon Louis, dominated the event. The entire stadium erupted in cheers as the winning runner easily beat his fellow competitors by a long lead. Thus, the modern marathon was firmly established.

The Infamous 26.2 Distance

When did the marathon become 26.2 miles? As Paul Smaras, a travel writer and promoter, points out with Jeff Galloway's help, "At the 1908 Olympic Games in London, the marathon distance was changed to twenty-six miles to cover the ground from Windsor Castle to White City stadium, with 385 yards added on so the race could finish in front of the royal family's viewing box. . . . After sixteen years of extremely heated discussion, this 26.2 mile distance was established at the 1924 Olympics in Paris as the official marathon distance."

The 26.2 mile distance is still run today. However, due to different cities hosting the Summer Olympics every four years, courses utilized for Olympic marathons can vary quite a bit (some are more hilly than others), therefore making it difficult to compare the performances of recent winners. Some Olympic marathons have been held in very hot and humid conditions as well. Men's and women's winning times for the Olympic marathons are a bit slower compared to other big-time marathons held around the world due in part to these events often being run in less than optimal weather conditions. Race strategy is often to win the race rather than run a fast time.

FACTS

The winner of the first Olympic and modern marathon was Spiridon Louis. He was a Greek postal worker. He won the event with a time of 2 hours, 58 minutes, 50 seconds. That's an average pace of 7:11 minutes per mile!

The Marathon Gains Notoriety

How the marathon gained notoriety as a single, individual event all on its own is another story. One of the runners in the marathon event in Athens in 1896 was Arthur Blake. Blake was sponsored by the Boston Athletic Association. Although he failed to finish the marathon, Blake medalled in another event and was considered a local hero. The Boston Athletic Club was so enamored of the long-run event that, on the boat trip back from Athens, they decided they would sponsor a similar event to commemorate the famous ride of Paul Revere in 1775. And so it was that the first official marathon in the United States was held on April 19, 1897. Eighteen runners were entered.

In 1898, the field of entrants grew to twenty-five and the crowds and news coverage was huge. By 1900, the craze was full blown and the Boston Athletic Association marathon's reputation was firmly established. Today's Boston Marathon is one of the country's premier events, for which runners must quality by completing a marathon in a particular time for their age group, typically under three-and-a-half hours. The field for 2001's Boston Marathon was 15,606 runners.

The now-defunct Yonkers marathon was actually the second marathon event established in the United States as an annual event. Today there are many marathons run all over the country at all times of year, one of the oldest being the Atlantic City Marathon. One of the most famous and the largest is the New York City Marathon, in which thousands of participants take part in each year. In was founded in the mid 1970s along with Chicago. Los Angeles joined the field in the mid-1980s. The Marine Corps

Marathon (held in Washington, D.C.) along with the Chicago Marathon, also attract huge fields in excess of 25,000 runners.

The Long Run: Cornerstone of the Marathon

Runners training to compete in a marathon must slowly and systematically build their distances of their long runs to a minimum of twenty miles. In fact, completing three runs of twenty to twenty-three miles in the ten weeks prior to the marathon are an important predictor of successfully completing the race.

The long run is also an important element for middle-distance runners. The recommended distance of the long run varies depending upon the experience and aspirations of the individual runner. The 10K runner will benefit from runs of eight miles, ten miles, and even up to fourteen miles or more. A 5K runner will benefit from runs of six miles, eight miles, and up to twelve miles or so.

The long run has been emphasized as the building block of training for over thirty years. Arthur Lydiard and many others have made it the base component of training programs for distance runners. All of today's programs, including Hal Higdon's and Jeff Galloway's, highlight the importance of the long run.

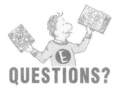

QUESTIONS?

What are the benefits of the long run?
The long run strengthens the heart, providing for a larger stroke volume; it strengthens the leg muscles critical for endurance; it develops mental toughness and coping skills; it increases fat burning capacity as well as capillary growth and myoglobin concentration into muscle fibers; and it increases aerobic efficiency.

Definition and Purposes of the Long Run

For the purposes of this discussion, the distance of a long run is considered to be ten miles and longer or a run that lasts over ninety minutes. It should be run approximately one minute slower than the pace you plan to run during the marathon. Or stated another way, the pace should be one to one-and-a-half minutes slower than your present 10K race pace. If your training schedule calls for a long run of eighteen miles, the distance must be run at one time rather than splitting the distance into an eight-mile morning session and an eight-mile evening run.

The long run is the most important component of marathon training because it teaches the body to both mentally and physically tackle the challenges presented in completing the 26.2 mile event. Physiologically, the body must learn to switch over to fat storage site energy reserves after the glycogen (fuel stores in the muscles, converted over from carbohydrate food sources) have been depleted. One must also be accustomed to running for very long periods of time, and the mental toughness that develops from completing long training runs pays off handsome dividends during the actual marathon.

Above all, marathon training schedules must be designed so that runners are rested prior to undertaking their long runs. A runner who completes two to three long runs of twenty miles or longer prior to his or her marathon will no doubt reduce the possibility of visiting the dreaded "wall" (the point in time when the glycogen stores in one's leg muscles become depleted and a runner's pace can slow down to a crawl).

The majority of runners who experience difficulty in completing their long training runs fail to prepare adequately for these critical workouts. So remember, both long runs and the marathon itself don't have to be painful experiences. The key is to plan ahead. See Chapter 12 for a discussion of how to prepare for running long.

ALERT

It is important to follow the hard/easy method of training we've discussed before. Pressing too hard without scheduled rest periods or reduced workloads more often than not will only lead to injuries and delays. Do not become obsessed with your training and run on what are supposed to be rest days. This approach can lead to injury, fatigue, and even burnout.

Making the Long Run Easier and Safer

Don't schedule long runs too early in your training, even if you are physically prepared to cover the distance. This may lead to staleness or premature burnout. Additionally, you may "peak" too early in your training. Also, schedule some long runs at the same time of day the actual marathon will be held to familiarize yourself with running during that time frame and to also develop a pre-race routine that you feel comfortable with.

Consider running for cumulative time, approximating the distance. Doing so will enable you to have more flexibility and spontaneity in regards to the route you choose to run. However, do your longest run no closer than three to four weeks before the marathon. The distance of this run should be twenty-three miles maximum. Above all, do not run 26.2 miles in practice to see if you can run a marathon. Save your efforts for the actual race!

Do not increase the distance of your long run by more than 10 percent per week. This equates to adding approximately fifteen minutes to each subsequent long run. Every fourth week, drop the distance of your long run, along with your total weekly mileage, providing for an easy week of training to facilitate rest and recovery.

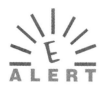

When training, think about running with others. Running with a group will make the long run more pleasurable and easier to accomplish as opposed to running alone. While running with a group is a great idea, be sure you don't turn long runs into races. This will almost surely lead to injury.

Areas of Experimentation

One beneficial aspect of marathon training that can't be overlooked is the opportunity to experiment with a variety of miscellaneous concerns (e.g., shoes, nutrition) prior to incorporating them in the actual 26.2-mile event. A cardinal rule of marathoning is: Don't try anything new on race day. In other words, don't leave anything to chance regarding the marathon. Use all training runs as opportunities for experimentation.

First, think about your shoes. Which type of shoes work best for you? Are you comfortable with the pair you are wearing? How much mileage is currently on them? Will you be able to train in them and still have both ample cushioning/support to absorb the shock your legs will experience during the marathon, keeping discomfort to a minimum while helping protect you from injury?

If your shoes are currently causing you any discomfort during training, you should not intend to use them for a marathon. Talk to a local professional at a specialty running store for advice on a different shoe to train and race in as soon as possible. You should decide upon a specific brand to wear for final long training run and, of course, for the marathon at least six weeks prior to the marathon.

Socks are also important. Which type of socks (e.g., thin, think, two layers, various materials, etc.) work best for you? There's no worse feeling in a marathon than realizing that your socks are causing blisters to develop at only the halfway point!

Additionally, consider all of your running apparel. What type of clothing won't cause chafing? How much and what type of clothing do you need to wear to be comfortable yet not become overheated (e.g., gloves, hat, long-sleeves)?

Beyond apparel, consider other things that may go on your body. For example, do you plan to use analgesic creams (e.g., Ben Gay, Myoflex, Sportscreme, etc.) during the marathon? Some experts claim that they can't penetrate deep enough to relieve muscular discomfort. Others say that creams are effective in reducing pain and inflammation. Similarly, what about Skin-Lube/Vaseline? Should you apply these products? If yes, how much and where should they be applied (e.g., under arms, toes, between legs, nipples, etc.)?

For your pre-race routine, consider what you are going to eat. Think about the pre-race evening meal, for instance. What type of carbohydrate meal do you crave (e.g., pasta, potatoes, rice, etc.)? What foods seem to give you the most energy? How much do you need to eat? Are there any foods that you should avoid so as not to cause digestive problems?

Similarly, how about the race morning snack? What type of foods work best for you, yielding both energy while at the same time not causing stomach discomfort or cramps? Should you partake in coffee or caffeine? If yes, how much should you drink and how soon before the marathon? Some research suggests that drinking caffeinated products spares glycogen early in a marathon. The flip side is that caffeine is a diuretic and thus may lead to dehydration. The bottom line is that if you choose to consume caffeine, be sure to also drink water to avoid dehydration.

ESSENTIALS   Many local honey makers and produce stores carry honey sticks, plastic straws filled with different flavored honeys. These are very easy to carry with you on long runs because they're small and lightweight.

Rest is as important as eating before a race. Figure out what time you need to retire to get a good night's sleep. Also, determine how early you need to rise to take care of everything you need to do, such as eating breakfast, hydrating, and visiting the bathroom.

During the race, you'll need to have a plan for hydration. How often do you need to drink during the marathon, and should you consume sports drinks or just water at every aid station? These are some very important questions that will need answers prior to your marathon.

Finally, decide whether or not you will rely on gels as a supplemental energy source during the marathon (as many runners do). There are many types of gels to choose from now. The key is finding the particular product that works for you. Training runs are great opportunities to decide how many packets you will need to consume during the marathon, when they should be taken (at what mile markers/elapsed marathon time), along with determining whether they will cause stomach discomfort.

ESSENTIALS   It is perfectly acceptable to come to a complete stop for one to two minutes to take time to drink fluids, stretch, hit the restroom, or whatever else you find necessary within a long run. Brief stops such as these will have no adverse effect on your preparedness to successfully complete the marathon.

Marathon Training Schedules

Before proceeding to your choice of the two marathon training schedules that follow, it is essential that you successfully complete a base-building period by utilizing one of the two mileage buildup scheduled featured in Chapter 5. It cannot be stressed enough that both of the marathon training schedules offered below are designed for runners who have successfully competed the mileage buildup period. If you have skipped weeks and/or did not complete the buildup phase, then do not proceed.

Additionally, it is very important that you have read the majority of the text contained within this book. Using a training schedule without basic knowledge of training principles and injury prevention strategies, or without the consultation of a coach or the advice of a knowledgeable/experienced runner, can indeed be hazardous to your health!

If you cannot complete the mileage specified for the first four weeks in these schedules without injury or resultant pain, then you should revisit the mileage buildup schedules. Scale back your training to a level that enables you to train safely without leg fatigue, soreness, and/or injury.

Schedule 1 (Beginner)

While this schedule features a bit less weekly mileage than the advanced marathon schedule (Schedule 2), runners who complete the workouts specified here will still be well-prepared to run 26.2 miles successfully on marathon day. Another attractive feature of this schedule is that it is based on a four-day training week, ideal for people faced with the demands of a busy work schedule, family commitments, and/or other obligations and responsibilities.

Schedule 2 (Advanced)

This is an eighteen-week program geared to the runner who completed the more advanced mileage buildup schedule that features higher weekly mileage. As with the beginner's schedule, you'll notice that this schedule builds up mileage gradually. In the first week you will run thirty-four miles for the week. You will gradually hit varying peaks in weeks six, eleven, and fourteen.

MARATHON TRAINING SCHEDULE 1 (BEGINNER)

WEEK #	SUN.	MON.	TUE	WED.	THUR.	FRI.	SAT.	TOTAL
1	10	Rest	5	Rest	5	Rest	4	24
2	5	Rest	4	Rest	4	Rest	4	17 LIGHT WEEK
3	11	Rest	5	Rest	6	Rest	4	26
4	12	Rest	6	Rest	6	Rest	4	28
5	13	Rest	6	Rest	7	Rest	4	30
6	6	Rest	4	Rest	4	Rest	4	18 LIGHT WEEK
7	15	Rest	7	Rest	7	Rest	4	33
8	17	Rest	7	Rest	8	Rest	4	36
9	19	Rest	7	Rest	9	Rest	4	39
10	7	Rest	4	Rest	4	Rest	4	19 LIGHT WEEK
11	21	Rest	7	Rest	9	Rest	4	41
12	14	Rest	7	Rest	10	Rest	4	35
13	8	Rest	4	Rest	4	Rest	4	20 LIGHT WEEK
14	22	Rest	7	Rest	9	Rest	4	42
15	12	Rest	7	Rest	10	Rest	4	33
16	14	Rest	7	Rest	5	Rest	4	30
17	10	Rest	6	Rest	4	Rest	Rest	20 LIGHT WEEK
18	26.2	Rest	Rest	Rest	Rest	Rest	Rest	MARATHON WEEK

MARATHON TRAINING SCHEDULE 2 (ADVANCED)

WEEK #	SUN.	MON.	TUES.	WED.	THUR.	FRI.	SAT.	TOTAL
1	10	Rest	6	8	6	Rest	4	34
2	12	Rest	6	8	6	Rest	4	36
3	6	Rest	4	Rest	4	Rest	4	18 LIGHT WEEK
4	14	Rest	6	8	6	Rest	4	38
5	16	Rest	6	8	6	Rest	5	41
6	18	Rest	6	8	6	Rest	5	43
7	6	Rest	5	Rest	5	Rest	4	20 LIGHT WEEK
8	20	Rest	5	7	6	Rest	4	42
9	14	Rest	6	8	6	Rest	4	38
10	7	Rest	5	Rest	6	Rest	4	22 LIGHT WEEK
11	21	Rest	5	7	6	Rest	4	43
12	14	Rest	6	8	6	Rest	4	38
13	8	Rest	6	Rest	6	Rest	4	24 LIGHT WEEK
14	22–23	Rest	5	7	6	Rest	5	45–46
15	12	Rest	6	8	6	Rest	4	36
16	14	Rest	7	Rest	5	Rest	4	30
17	10	Rest	6	Rest	4	Rest	1–2 Opt.	20–22 TAPER WEEK
18	26.2	Rest	Rest	Rest	Rest	Rest	Rest	MARATHON WEEK

Mentally Training for the Marathon

In this section, a variety of mental strategies will be discussed that will enable you to set realistic goals, complete the necessary training (in particular, the long runs), and be optimally prepared mentally for the challenges that await you in completing the marathon.

FACTS

Some of the techniques you can use to psyche yourself up both during marathon training and the actual races include mental rehearsal/visualization (creating pictures in your mind), imagery (playing out/imagining the way you wish for an event to occur), and self-talk (giving yourself positive affirmations).

Before You Begin

There are certain "prerequisites" or internal characteristic that a runner must possess in order to undertake the necessary training that a marathon requires. These include motivation, self-discipline, and effective time-management, all of which are characteristics that are interrelated. While a coach can provide interest and enthusiasm regarding the training program he or she designs and presents, motivation and self-discipline must be developed primarily from within.

The best marathon training program in the world will not enable a runner to make it to the finish line of a marathon if he or she isn't internally motivated to undergo and complete the training and then finish the race. By the same token, it requires a great deal of self-discipline to complete the long training runs while coping with other daily distractions and managing all the personal responsibilities of daily life. This is why it is crucial that the runner who wishes to train for the marathon be an effective manager of time.

Short- and Long-Term Goal Setting

For most first-time marathoners, goal setting is simple: They just want to finish the race. However, beyond that basic goal, there are other types of goals that can be set in order to help enrich the marathon experience. There are two basic types of goals: process goals and outcome goals. It is important to set short-term objectives (process goals) on your way to achieving the big goal (outcome goal).

Process goals are types of goals involving activities that focus on mastering the task and increasing one's skill level (such as the knowledge and training needed to complete a marathon). Examples of process goals include following the training schedule as closely as possible; improving your nutrition; reading as much as you can about the marathon; consulting with your coach on a regular basis; and getting more sleep to be as rested as possible.

On the other hand, outcome goals relate to the finished product; they're the goals you hope to accomplish in the marathon. Examples include breaking four hours in the marathon; running the second half of the marathon faster than the first 13.1 miles; defeating a rival; and running a personal best in the marathon.

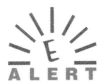
ALERT

When selecting goals, it is best to be as specific as possible. Be sure to write the goals down, perhaps tell others about your goals, and set a time frame for achieving the goals. These strategies will enhance the possibility of achieving both your short-term objectives as well as your big goals.

In the weeks prior to the marathon, think about three outcome goals you'd be interested in accomplishing for your race: an easily obtainable goal, a realistic yet moderately challenging goal, and an ultimate goal. Determine a strategy to achieve the ultimate goal, but build in flexibility in your plan to shoot for less ambitious goals if things don't pan out the way you had planned. Above all, be realistic. For example, if you aren't genetically gifted to run a sub thirty-eight minute 10K, there's very little chance you will be able to break three hours in the marathon.

Strategies for Completing the Training

Finding someone to guide you and to encourage you can be a great help. If possible, find a coach who has a reputation for being both enthusiastic and possesses a positive attitude. These traits can help inspire and motivate you. Or join a group or team whose members share your same goals. These individuals can provide the needed emotional support. Groups or a training partner can help make completing the long runs easier than doing these alone. It is essential to find people who run your approximate pace so that long runs do not turn into races.

When running long, break the course into sections mentally. That is, mentally run from one landmark to the next instead of thinking of the entire twenty-mile training course as a single entity. When you reach the first landmark, then mentally think of running to the next and so forth.

Realize that the training will not always be easy. If running a marathon were simple, there would be no challenge as everyone would be able to do it. To enable you to cope with the physical and mental demands of completing the long training runs and the actual marathon when the going gets tough, there are several mental strategies you can utilize.

Examples of Mental Strategies

Here are three different tools for mental preparation to help combat some of the difficulties of the long run. They will all come in handy and are quite effective.

Self-Talk Thoughts

Talking to yourself is easy, yet it is very effective in keeping yourself on track. Here are some phrases you might try saying to yourself:

- "If this was easy, then everybody could complete a marathon."
- "Keep running . . . maybe I'll feel better when I have some Gatorade."
- "If I quit now, I'll be very disappointed in myself later this afternoon."

- "I'm not really physically tired, I'm more fatigued mentally."
- "Completing this important training run will give me confidence and enable me to finish the marathon comfortably."
- "In just one more hour, this run will be finished and I'll be at home showering, relaxing, eating, etc."

Imagery

Imagine situations in which you are succeeding at what you do, and it will become a reality. For example, imagine that you are a world-class marathoner and in the lead of the Boston or Olympic Marathon. Imagine that your running form is smooth and graceful. Imagine that you are running effortlessly and very relaxed. You'll be surprised at how this technique can help you!

Visualization/Mental Rehearsal Strategies

Like imagery, visualization is a great way to see yourself accomplishing your goal and making it happen. Try some of these visualizations. Picture yourself running every mile of the marathon for which you are training. Visualize what the finish line area will look like (for instance, with the clock displaying the time you're shooting for). See in your "mind's eye" the spectators who will be cheering for you. Think of all your friends back home who will be pulling for you while you are running.

The Week Before the Marathon

As you taper (which will be discussed shortly), concentrate on reading books and magazine articles that will provide you with motivation and inspiration. Take care of any anxieties and concerns in the weeks prior to the marathon. Preparation is the best strategy to reduce or eliminate stress and anxiety. That's all the more reason to have completed those key long runs in the weeks prior to the marathon. Similarly, getting a head start on packing if traveling out of town is another way to reduce your stress level.

Remember that it is normal to be tense or nervous prior to a marathon. Even the most seasoned runners experience these feelings. Stay away from participants who are excessively stressed out or are negative so that these individuals can't adversely affect your state of mind.

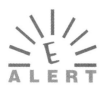

It's not always a good idea to view the course prior to the race. Doing so may add to your nervousness (particularly if the course is difficult). Instead, look at a course map and/or elevation profile diagram to become familiar with the characteristics of the course.

Preparing for Psychological Issues During the Marathon

If you've trained properly, and barring any unforeseen problems, nothing should stop you from achieving your goal of finishing the marathon. Nothing, that is, except a lack of confidence and/or a negative attitude at the starting line or during the race. When you line up at the starting line, don't just think that you can do it, *know* that you will finish.

As mentioned previously, finishing a marathon is seldom easy (for most participants). However, a positive mental attitude will go a long way in helping you finish with a smile on your face. Nothing builds confidence more than the long training runs (twenty miles and longer) that you will have completed in practice and that will enable you to know that you can finish the race.

ESSENTIALS

While you're out on the course, take time to enjoy the spectators, participants, and the scenery of the course; stop negative thoughts dead in their tracks and change them to positive affirmations; think about how proud family members and friends will be of you.

Tapering

Tapering is one of the steps you'll begin in the two weeks just before a race. You'll notice in the marathon training schedules that Week 17 is the taper week. The idea is to slow down. Less is best! Give your body the rest it will need to prepare for the big event. Do not use this time to get in extra exercise. Your body needs to be loose and rested.

Keep stretching in the couple of weeks prior to the marathon as much as possible. Consider getting a leg massage no more than two days before the marathon, but if you've never had a leg massage, don't try it now! Take care of long toenails, blisters, and calluses the week or two prior to the marathon.

Nutritional Issues the Week Before Your Marathon

As you scale back on the distance and intensity of your running during the last week, realize that you will not be burning as many calories. Therefore, you may gain one or two pounds if you don't cut back a bit on the quantity of your servings early in the week. Use care in selecting foods to eat during this time period, aiming for quality foods rather than snacks and high-fat products.

Carbohydrate loading begins three days before the marathon. Choose foods for lunch and dinner that are high in carbohydrates (such as pasta, potatoes, rice, and so on). Don't neglect fruits, vegetables, and some protein sources. Try to really scale back on fats during this time.

Hydrate well the week before the marathon (water is best) and, in particular, during the carbohydrate loading period (three days prior to the marathon). Research has shown that carbohydrates convert to glycogen more effectively when paired with the consumption of water. As mentioned above, this is the time when you may gain a couple of pounds, but don't worry about it. This is some of the fuel you will use during your marathon!

If you are traveling out of town, be sure to pack healthy snack foods you may wish to eat the weekend of the marathon. Eliminate the need to search for a grocery store that stocks your favorite foods. If traveling by plane to your marathon destination, carry bottled water with you. Flying at high altitudes causes dehydration.

A Beginning Marathoner's Story

Sometimes it helps to hear others' experiences to psyche you up for a challenge. Here's a personal account of running a first marathon to get you in the right frame of mind:

I've been running on and off (mostly off) for the past fifteen years, primarily as a means of staying in shape. The lack of consistency in my training was driven by my lack of motivation. I always ran alone and used the time to refresh my mind, but I had no external motivating influences or goals. Then, in the summer of 1998, an acquaintance told me about his "quest" to get into the NYC Marathon and all the preparation and training required to successfully complete a marathon. I was immediately intrigued with the idea of running 26 miles, 385 yards, and we continued to talk about running and what it takes to train for a marathon. After a beer or two or three my addictive personality kicked in and I knew I had to run a marathon. That day I made a commitment to complete a marathon before my fortieth birthday.

That conversation was the catalyst I needed to start running again. I had a long-term goal of completing a marathon, but I needed short-term goals to keep me motivated along the way. So I started entering 5Ks and 10Ks almost every weekend. There's nothing like the camaraderie and excitement on race day. These short runs were good but I needed to start doing long runs. But how long? How fast? How frequent? I knew if I was going to have the mental and physical conditioning required I needed some coaching.

The advice I got from Art Liberman's Web site (State of the Art Marathon Training at www.marathontraining.com*) regarding* these peripheral aspects of preparation gave me the additional confidence and correct state of mind going into my first marathon.

While my primary objective was to finish without pain or injury, it is also important to have stretch objectives and some emotional objectives as well. My additional objectives were: Finish under four hours, have fun, raise money for ALS, and have my family "participate" with me. I am happy to say I achieved them all.

The tips I received from Art during the weeks leading up to race day regarding planning, packing, traveling, tapering, hydration, nutrition, and stretching helped tremendously. I knew I had trained enough, but I was still nervous and stressed. Knowing I had the secondary training and planning elements covered relieved me of that burden and worry. One of the best pieces of planning was mapping out the route and the approximate times I would be passing certain mile marks. We had pre-planned where along the coarse we would "meet" and it worked out great. It sure beat just seeing me at the start, then waiting close to four hours for me to finish.

I felt good going into mile twenty-three, but by the end of twenty-three, I had hit my wall. The demons in my head were telling me to STOP NOW! But I used some self-talk coaching tips, which helped battle the little voices in my head. As I approached the finish line the feeling was overwhelming. People I didn't even know, along with a few I did know, cheering for me. The months of preparation, training, and support of my family paid off, I finished my first marathon in 3.55:20 (net). The emotional rush was awesome.

I'm now getting back into a routine, with my sights set on the New York City 2001 Marathon in November. I'm in!

—John Arminio, Montville, NJ

CHAPTER 17

The Marathon Experience

I n the previous chapter you learned about the marathon and how to train for it. This chapter is about the day or two before the marathon—final preparations and then running the race itself. This includes strategies, precautions, what to expect, and what to do when it's over.

Mental Preparation

If you're training for your first marathon and you've gotten this far, excellent! Are you convinced you're going to hit the wall at mile twenty-three and not be able to finish? Do you feel like your training has been going so well that you'll be able to finish the race in under three-and-a-half hours? Reality is somewhere in between. If you've been training according to this book and the advice you've sought from other runners and, possibly, a coach, then you're almost guaranteed to finish the marathon, whether you beat your time goal or not.

To inspire you for the event of your lifetime, here's what Shelley Barineau of Houston, Texas, said about her first marathon, the 2001 Compaq Houston Marathon:

> *I DID IT!!!! My race was fabulous. I was so prepared and had a lot of energy. The start was something I will never forget. Thousands of people like a wave for the first few miles, everyone excited and chatting. I hung back and ran about twelve minute miles for the first four. Then I picked it up and ran about 10:00 miles until mile twenty-three (including restroom breaks and, of course, stops for sports drinks at every aid station).*
>
> *I had so much energy at mile eighteen when I saw my family and friends, I knew I would finish. At mile twenty-three, I kicked it in and ran about nine-minute miles to the finish. I probably passed 250–300 people. I was smiling and feeling great. My family was at the finish.*
>
> *I accomplished a life-long dream. In life I have learned that if I give my best, I will be successful. Part of giving my best in this race was the advice and counsel of my coach, Art Liberman. Without his, my race would have been much different. Thanks, Art!*

Everyone's experience is unique. Everyone's experience is special. One thing's for sure, it's an experience you'll never forget. So let's see what you need to do to make the most of it.

Physical Preparation

After training so intensely for so long, you're going to feel like you're salvaging everything by not continuing to work hard the week before the marathon. But listen up: Don't! Stick to your schedule and taper as indicated.

This doesn't mean you want to be completely inactive or overeat the week before the race. It's a good idea to stretch as much as possible, always remembering to first warm up those muscles. In the week prior to the race, take some brisk walks or do some light cycling—but nothing that's going to strain your legs, just something to keep the blood flowing and endorphins up.

On a similar note, if you are traveling to an exciting destination for your marathon and planning on doing some sightseeing by foot, do so two days or more prior to the race. If your time is more limited, refrain from taking long walks the day prior to the marathon. Instead, do your sightseeing from the window of a tour bus or car to conserve your energy for the race.

Packing for an Out-of-Town Marathon

For out-of-town events in particular, don't wait until the night before you travel to collect and pack needed items. Rather, make a list of things you wish to take and begin getting them together in the days prior to departure.

Also, pin your race number to the front of your singlet or T-shirt. It's a good idea to take some toilet paper with you to the race site in case there's none remaining when you visit the bathroom or port-o-let. You'll have enough on your mind race morning, let alone worrying about items you need to wear or take to the starting line.

Check the weather forecast for the area the marathon will be run the day or two prior to the race. Plan for all possible types of weather conditions and pack accordingly. It's better to have everything you need rather than having to scurry around a new city looking for clothing and/or accessories at the last minute.

If you're traveling to an out-of-town race by air, your running shoes and apparel for the marathon should be packed in carry-on luggage so that should your baggage get lost or be delayed by the airline, you will at least have the "essential" items needed for the race.

Keep in mind that this list is not all-inclusive. Factors such as weather conditions, food preferences, etc. are quite variable. Try to allow for all contingencies:

- **Clothing**: singlet*, shorts*, sports bra*, socks*, shoes*, gloves**, hat**, T-shirt (long and short sleeve)**, sweat shirt**, tights**, warm-ups (jacket and long pants)**
- **Other handy items**: running watch, Vaseline or skin lube, foot powder, handkerchief, shoe laces, small gym bag, lock for locker, towel, race confirmation (to receive race number, if applicable), Ibuprofen, safety pins, sweat bands, analgesic creams (e.g., Ben Gay, Myoflex, etc.)
- **Possible food items***: Power Bars, gel supplements (e.g., GU, ReLode, etc.), snack items (e.g., bagels, whole grain muffins, honey sticks, fruit, etc.), carbo-load sports drinks, bottled water (especially for the airplane)

*If traveling to the race by air, pack these as carry-on luggage. Many runners have been left stranded in the past because shoes and socks were packed inside luggage that was delayed or lost by the airline.

**Optional items to wear prior to or during the marathon. Consider bringing some clothing that you can discard during the race after you warm up. Many people decorate or write on their T-shirts to make them more visible to family members who will be looking for them in the crowd, and to make it easier for spectators to cheer them on. You could try anything from your name to the name of your running club, your town, an organization you want to support, whatever. Be creative! You'll see all sorts of things on the other runners.

***Be sure that you have experimented with these or any other food items as part of your pre-race diet prior to the marathon.

Other Travel Considerations

Depending on how far you're traveling to the marathon, make sure you get there in plenty of time. Again, allow for possible airline or traffic delays so you don't feel rushed. If you're traveling to another time zone, particularly one with a time difference of more than one hour, give yourself time to arrive and acclimate.

The same holds true for traveling to a race that will be run in an environment significantly different from the one you're used to training in. For example, if you live in Maine and you're running a December marathon in Hawaii, try to arrive there at least a week prior to the race to acclimate somewhat to the higher temperature and humidity you'll be experiencing during the race. If you've been training for the past month or two in cool to cold temperatures and will be running a marathon that will be held in significantly warmer conditions, arriving one to two days prior to the event will not be adequate time for your body to acclimate.

Acclimating to heat and humidity takes a minimum of a week or even longer. If you've trained properly in cool conditions by completing all your scheduled workouts, you'll still be able to finish the marathon; however, the keys to success in this situation will be to set conservative rather than highly competitive goals and by running the race at a slower pace than if the event were held in your home town.

Try to find a hotel close to the start and finish of the race. If they're all beyond your budget, already booked, or you want to stay with a friend or family in the area, map out how you're going to get to the start in plenty of time. Remember, too, you get what you pay for most times. Better yet, drive to the race start location the day before to make sure you know the best roads to take to get there and where you will park. Oftentimes, roads near the course will be closed the day of the marathon, thus limiting your access to the start of the race.

Be sure to carefully read all the race literature prior to the event so as to familiarize yourself with all aspects of the event (documentation you need (such as a photo ID to obtain your race number, road closures, start and finish line procedures, location of aid stations/portable toilets, shuttle bus schedules, to name just a few). Don't assume that the starting line of the event will be set up adjacent to where marathon race headquarters was located the day prior (where registration and the expo is often held) as you will be in for a big shock!

You're going to be nervous enough the night before and morning of the race that you probably won't want to socialize much, even with your family. You'll want to retire early, taking your mind off the race until the next morning. Your peace of mind may necessitate spending the extra money for the convenience of a hotel located near the start of the race at least for the night before the race. Plan to stay with friends or family the night following the race; you'll want to celebrate then, anyway.

The Evening Prior to Your Marathon

Be sure to eat carbohydrate products that have been "tried and proven" during your training period. Keep pasta sauces simple, avoiding high-fat varieties (e.g., alfredo, pesto, and so on). Avoid eating lots of salad items and vegetables (roughage) as these may prove to be troublesome on race day and cause digestive problems. Stick to water before, during, and after the evening meal. Try to consume eight ounces at least every half-hour. Because coffee and tea contain caffeine, drinking them the night before the race may make it difficult for you to fall asleep easily.

After your meal, try not to think about the marathon any more that evening. Instead, watch television, read (about something other than running), or find something else restful to do until turning in for the evening.

Prior to retiring, have two alarm systems set to wake you up (alarm clock, wake-up call, running watch alarm setting, whatever works). While this may seem compulsive for some people, the key here is not leaving anything to chance.

Wake up early enough to eat appropriately, make a visit to the bathroom, and take care of anything you feel the need to do so as not to feel rushed. The few hours before the marathon is a time to relax and stay focused as much as possible.

The Pre-Race Morning

To take some of the time and worry out of having to think of all this stuff yourself, here's a checklist of things to think about that's been devised from experience:

As mentioned previously, wake up early enough to take care of everything you must do (eat and drink, visit the bathroom, dress, and so on). If you haven't already done so, have a plan to meet your family members or friends at a designated time and place after the race. Being specific regarding location is particularly important if the marathon you will be running has several thousand people in its entry field! Have a backup plan if for some reason you are unable to meet at a predetermined time and location after the race.

Check the weather forecast again for updated information about conditions, temperature range, and wind. Having this information helps in deciding what you may choose to wear for the majority of the marathon. Above all, don't overdress.

Finally, leave for the race site with plenty of time to spare, arriving early enough to check your bag (if necessary) and take care of any last-minute details. Stay off your feet as much as possible prior to the race. Continue to drink fluids up to fifteen minutes before the start of the race. Eat your final snack no more than thirty minutes before the start of the race.

During the Marathon

Runners will start lining up about fifteen minutes before the starting time. Line up according to your expected pace (faster runners to the front). In a large race the slower runners can actually create problems (as people tend to be pushed down or slip and fall). Please be courteous!

Also, don't get too caught up in the hoopla by being overly exuberant and yelling and cheering as the gun is about to go off. Save that energy for later when you'll need it. Instead, focus on positive thinking. Visualize all of your friends who will be pulling for you and all the hard training that went into the preparation for this big race. Take a deep breath and know that you are going to not only finish the race but achieve your goals.

Pacing

Running the correct pace for your ability level is crucial in the marathon, especially for the first time marathoner. It is so easy to start the race running much faster than you had originally planned to do or should. Your pace during the first mile often feels effortless due to the adrenaline rush and excitement of the event. If you go out too fast, you'll pay dearly for the mistake in the later miles.

A much better strategy is to start out slower than what you hope to average and then run the middle miles at your chosen (hopefully realistic) pace. It's a better strategy to pick up the pace during the final miles when you know you can finish rather than starting aggressively. In the world of marathoning, there's no such theory as "putting the fast miles in the bank early in the race" and then holding on in the end. If you go that route, you will most assuredly visit the dreaded wall.

Also take into consideration weather conditions and course difficulty in predicting your possible marathon times. Strong winds, high temperatures, and hills can add several minutes to your finish time. During the marathon, monitor how you are feeling constantly, and adjust your pace accordingly based on your perceived energy level. Your past long training runs will provide you with the experience that will enable you to do this. Here's how Ben Bobrow, an emergency room physician from Las Vegas, Nevada, described his experience:

The training program really worked! I was feeling really strong at the beginning of the race, but just kept thinking about taking it easy at the beginning. I ran in a pack of about five to seven guys from miles ten to eighteen or so. I kept thinking to myself, some of us should not be here at this pace (6:25) but I was not sure if it was ME that should not be there. I kept slowing down to take drinks, and ate some gels, and they were drinking water and sometimes skipping stations, and no gels, but I kept catching up to them each mile, and I kept thinking, at mile twenty I will be ready to roll, and sure enough at mile twenty, the other guys started dropping like flies and I was doing pretty well, and just tried to keep the same pace. I passed a lot of people the last six miles, and finished strongly. I felt fine after the race. In retrospect the whole program worked out great, no injuries, I did not waste a lot of time training improperly and had a good race and felt good afterwards. I really could not have asked for more!

Aid Stations

Do not pass up any fluid station. While it's okay to drink just water in the early miles, runners must consume sports beverages no later than sixty minutes of running (and earlier if desired). Find out what works best for you in long practice runs.

Water is usually offered at the first tables at an aid station with sports beverages served near the end of the station. If you're not sure what's in the cup (water or sports drink), politely ask. It's not a good feeling splashing what you think is water on your head or chest to cool off and discovering a second or two later that the cool liquid is actually a sports drink!

Here's a tried and proven method for drinking on the go: Squeeze the top of the cup into a "v" shape to create a smooth delivery of fluid directly into your mouth if you choose to run and drink through the aid stations. If you haven't mastered the fine art of drinking while on the run or prefer an alternate approach, it's perfectly fine to walk through the aid stations to be sure that you are able to consume the entire contents of the cup. If you decide to stop and drink, please step to the side so as not to block other runners' access to the aid tables or race course.

Supplementing

Many runners now are taking advantage of the energy gel products available to endurance athletes on the go. These products provide a fairly quick source of carbohydrates (energy). Be sure you chase these products down with water to avoid stomach cramps and to insure absorption. Some runners will stop and eat a power bar, orange slices, jelly beans, etc. to also provide needed energy. These products are seldom offered at "official" marathon aid stations. As always, experiment in practice during your long runs with any food products you plan to eat during the marathon.

To Socialize or Not?

Chances are that during the marathon you will encounter other runners who will be running your pace and may wish to engage you in conversation. It is a personal decision whether you wish to stick with them and chat along the way. The positive aspect of socializing is that many great friendships have been started this way, and that talking to others is a great way to take your mind off the physical discomfort you may face later in the marathon. If both runners are experiencing great difficulty later in the event, pacts are often made to provide the necessary motivation for each runner to finish.

The other view is that talking may rob you of valuable energy you'll need later. The last miles of the marathon can be quite draining mentally. For that reason itself, you may choose to run the last miles without much conversation. Also, running with someone may slow you down. You'll undoubtedly finish the marathon, but sticking with someone who is slower may compromise your chances of achieving a goal you set for yourself.

On the Course

Once the race is underway, think pacing and overall goals. Remember what you set out to do and monitor yourself so you have the greatest chance to succeed. You will no doubt be buoyed by the energy of the other runners around you, and of the spectators along the course. Tap into it and let it carry you along but don't get overzealous and run too fast at first. Be grateful. Doesn't it feel good to be alive, good to be in the actual race, geared up to do 26.2?

If you feel an increase in pain as you continue to run, seriously consider dropping out of the marathon. No race is worth the risk of hurting yourself by continuing to run and causing a minor injury to turn into a major setback.

If you've never run a marathon, there is no way to truly describe or fully understand what special feelings you will be experiencing during the event. Savor and enjoy each and every moment. Take in all the sites and sounds along the way. High-five the extended hand of a child who views you as an athlete competing at center court. Smile at the spectator telling you "You're looking strong." Offer some brief words of encouragement to a fellow runner who may not be feeling as strong as you are. Enjoy the diverse scenery along the race course whether it be from a bridge you will be crossing, a hill affording a panoramic view of the countryside, or store fronts while cruising down main street. These are just some of the memories that you will experience along with the accomplishment of goal you worked so hard to achieve.

Immediately Following the Marathon

Right after you finish running, do the following:

- After crossing the line and turning in the stub on your race number, index card handed to you, or computer chip (each marathon has its own finish line record-keeping system), get something to drink.
- Determine if you have a need to visit the medical tent; blisters and excessive pain to muscles and joints should be checked out by the medical personnel on hand.
- Within a few minutes of finishing, grab something to eat.
- Stretch thoroughly within twenty minutes of finishing.
- Do not even consider lying down: Keep walking.
- Sign up for a post-race massage (if available).

After you return home or to the hotel, have a nice lunch. This should be a well-balanced meal that includes the majority of its total calories in carbohydrates. Don't overlook consuming at least 20 percent of the total calories from protein sources.

Do not take a nap or lay down for long periods of time (that is unless you wish to be very sore or nauseous). Instead, stay on your feet by taking a walk or perhaps going for an easy bike ride of a few miles. Above all, keep moving to minimize leg muscle soreness.

Later that afternoon or evening, go out and celebrate. If you trained properly and followed all of the pre-race and marathon strategy suggestions, you should be able to do just about anything you wish (including dancing!). Above all, have a great time.

Post-Marathon Evaluation

The marathon is a mystical event because so many factors come into play in determining how well you do and how much discomfort you will experience. Did you experience the infamous "wall"? With the marathon behind you, it's now time to think about the things you did correctly along with errors you may have made in your training and racing. Below is a list of some evaluation questions you might want to consider in assessing your total marathon experience, both training for and participating in the event. If necessary, modify and adjust your program to address these issues the next time you train for a marathon.

It's important to reflect upon what you might have done better and what you might have done differently if you had the chance. If you have any desire to run another marathon, which many do, you'll want to make the next one easier and more successful than your previous one.

Marathon Report Card Checklist

You should review how the marathon went for you by considering the following: Did you train smart and make it to the starting line healthy and injury-free? Did you avoid injury throughout your training enabling you to complete most of your scheduled workouts? Did you listen to your body and make minor adjustments to your training schedule thus becoming stronger and not worn down?

Think also about your training and how it contributed to your performance. Did you train consistently? Did you complete most of the scheduled workouts? Above all, did you complete all or most of your long runs (18–22/23 milers)?

Evaluate your race strategies. Did you eat and drink properly before, during, and after the marathon (and long training runs)? Did you run the correct pace for your present ability and conditioning level during the marathon (and long training runs)? Did you make adjustments for unforeseen problems (e.g., blisters, chafing, stomach discomfort, muscle cramps, etc.) during the marathon (and long training runs)? Completing the scheduled long runs and experimenting with a variety of issues will decrease the chances of incurring blisters, chafing, miscellaneous cramps during the marathon.

Finally, think about your mental approach to the marathon. Did you have the best possible mental/psychological attitude during the marathon (and throughout your training)? Were your marathon goals realistic?

Staying Motivated and Combating Burnout

It is not uncommon for runners to experience varying degrees of post-event depression (the blahs, decreased motivation, etc.) after finishing a marathon. This is due in part to achieving a goal that took much time and energy. Now that the goal has been accomplished, runners can sometimes feel a void in their lives. Until you are ready both mentally and physically to set new goals, consider the following strategies to deal with reduced motivation and/or burnout: Run simply for fun, not worrying about following a training schedule; supplement your running by participating in cross-training activities; take a break from running altogether; spend more time with family and friends and enjoy some social activities or nonathletic hobbies.

Life after the Marathon

After experiencing the personal satisfaction of completing one's first marathon, many runners are interested in returning to their training immediately. While completing a marathon is quite exciting and motivating, extreme care must be taken in the weeks and months following the event regarding rebuilding mileage to pre-marathon levels. The effects on the musculoskeletal system are significant as muscles have undergone micro-trauma, a fancy word for very small tears of the muscle tissue that normally occurs as a result of the physical demands of the marathon. These muscular tears require adequate time to heal and regenerate. Jumping right into a heavy training schedule will slow down the recovery of muscles and soft-connective tissue.

Even if the micro-trauma damage to the muscles is minimal, ligaments, joints, and bones are in a vulnerable state immediately following the marathon. To reduce the possibility of causing an injury, a prudent approach to the full resumption of training should be taken.

Some texts state that runners should take a couple of weeks off with no running after a marathon. Instead, it is recommended to engage in cross-training activities to maintain cardiovascular fitness while at the same time allowing the body to heal. Listen to your body and don't push it! If your body tells you that it needs more time to recover, by all means give it the rest that it needs.

You should view the next four to six weeks as a reverse taper. No running for the first week will help you recover more than light running. The next week you'll do some light runs and build it back up over the subsequent weeks. Eat healthy. A high carbohydrate diet in the first few days will help replenish your depleted carbs, and protein will help to rebuild damaged muscle tissue. Soups, juices, breads, and other healthy food will probably taste great too.

With lots of sleep and some easy walks, you'll be ready to run again in no time. Remember that the basic recovery process takes about a month, and during this time you will have to continue to rest, run easy, avoid speed work, and keep your carbohydrate load high. The rule of one day of recovery for each mile raced, or perhaps one day for each kilometer raced for masters runners and novices, is a rule you should really follow. The marathon was 26.2 miles or approximately 42.2 kilometers. Make sure you take the time to properly recover. If you are having serious pain, more than the usual post-marathon aches and pains, you should visit a sports medicine specialist.

Scheduling Your Next Marathon

If you have performed well in one marathon, be careful not to run and race too soon because you are at a high risk for injury during the next six to eight weeks. Running another marathon, a fast 10K, or ten-miler, or deciding to do another twenty-mile training run, etc., between marathons that are spaced too close together could be enough to cause a lingering injury.

So how long should you wait before doing your next marathon? The answer to that question depends on lots of factors. Some of these include, but are not limited to, years of running experience, type/intensity of the training program utilized for the previous marathon, energy/effort expended during that marathon, and duration/completeness of leg recovery from the previous marathon.

Most experts say that two marathons should be the limit one should run per year (spaced six months apart). This rule applies both to the novice (regardless of marathon pace) along with the advanced runner who turns in a competitive (maximal) effort.

Experienced runners who complete their previous marathon at a moderate to easy effort may be able to compete in another 26.2-mile race sooner than the recommended six-month waiting period. How much sooner depends upon the factors mentioned in the previous paragraph.

The central concept to consider is that the body needs adequate time to recover from a marathon. Training for and competing in another before one's legs have fully recovered can lead to a variety of overuse injuries. Is it worth the risk? The decision is ultimately yours. Good luck with your upcoming marathons!

CHAPTER 18

What's Next? Ultra-Running!

While the name or phrase ultra-marathoning may be more familiar to you, today's extra long-distance runners refer to themselves as ultra-runners. One thing for sure, it's a really far way to run.

Ultra-Running Basics

As if 26.2 miles wasn't quite far enough, ultra-marathoning is something that is becoming more and more popular. Ultra-marathon events are usually either 50 or 100 miles. There is also the 100K, which is sixty-two miles. However, there are some that are more than 100 miles in a given event. The most popular ultra-marathons average about 100 miles. There are also twenty-four-hour events. All in all, the world of ultra-marathoning is quite varied. According to David Blaikie, an ultra-runner and writer, "Ultra races typically begin at fifty kilometers and can extend to enormous distances. There is no limit."

Nick Marshall, in the last chapter of his book, *The Complete Marathon*, wrote, "In any endurance activity like distance running, there will always be a fringe group interested in pushing the limits further. It is the nature of the beast to seek new tests when the proportions of the old ones have lost their capacity to inspire awe."

But of course that still doesn't answer the question, "Why?" Marshall's response: "To question why anyone would want to venture beyond that barrier is merely to rehash the perplexing and ultimately personal question of why we run in the first place. Why not?"

This section is a brief introduction to the world of ultra-running. Here, and in the resources section, you will find all the information you need to satisfy your interest or begin a new running life if this sounds like something you would enjoy.

The History of the Ultra-Marathon

Long-distance runs such as these are not new. In fact, at the turn of the last century, long-distance runs of this nature were the norm. The marathon was an obscure distance. Many regions of the nation watched competitions between amateur and professional athletes in races that lasted well more than five days. Many of the nation's great runners of the 1800s ran more than fifty miles in most events.

Races across America were not uncommon. In fact, until the Great Depression in the 1930s, it was not unusual to see stories in newspapers of another athlete claiming to have broken the national record for traversing the continent. And this was done in the time when training techniques and our understanding of biomechanics were still not thought of.

Add to that the fact that these individuals were not running in anything that approximates today's running shoes, let alone sneakers. They ran in leather shoes! Sneakers didn't even exist. Nor did sports drinks, gel energy supplements, high-tech fabrics, 100-lap sports watches, heart rate monitors, or other products that we take for granted today.

Long-distance running like ultra-running didn't become popular until the mid-1970s and early '80s. One of the leaders in this movement was Ted Corbitt, who was an Olympian and a running enthusiast. He often went to the London-Brighton double marathon, and urged many clubs in the United States to sponsor such events. Slowly, the New York City Road Runners Club gave in and sponsored a few races.

Out west it was a little different. In 1974 a race was held—a horse race. The race was in California, and the course started in Squaw Valley and went all the way to Auburn. The distance was 100 miles. Gordie Ainsleigh completed the race running the entire course without a horse! This was the beginning of one of the most famous ultra-marathons in the world today, the Western States 100.

In reality, the first organized ultra-marathon was held in the Midwest in 1970. Today there are hundreds of ultra-marathons around the country and many more around the world.

Organizers of Ultra-Running

The world of the ultra-runners is highly organized with international governing bodies, national organizations, and many clubs. The IAU is the International Association of Ultra-Runners. American Ultra-Running Association (AUA) is the United States branch of that organization. These organizations develop the rules and policies that most of the popular and legitimate events abide by.

The AUA is also a member of the USA Track & Field (USATF). The AUA claims it is not a governing body, and issues no rules, but abides by many other rules outlined by more world-renowned organizations. The goal of the AUA is "to keep its focus on communication, development, and promotion of the sport, maximizing administrative efficiency."

Ultra-Running Events

The events in ultra-running vary greatly. The types of races and the way winners are determined are not always the same from race to race. To be sure, the winners of some of the shorter ultra-marathons, such as the fifty-mile races, are determined just like the popular distance races from the mile to the marathon. First to cross the finish line wins. However, the ultra-runners can be much more imaginative

As Blaikie writes, "The longest certified ultra-marathon in the world is The Ultimate Ultra, the annual Sri Chinmoy 1,300-Miler (2,092 kilometers), which is held each fall in New York." In the famous New York one-mile loop, Sri Chinmoy runners circle the course 1,300 times. "There is also the annual Trans America Footrace, which is run in sixty-four consecutive daily stages from Los Angeles to New York. Runners cover almost 3,000 miles (more than 4,800 kilometers) at a rate of about 45 miles (72 kilometers) a day."

FACTS

In the ultra-marathoning world, there is a series of races, known as the Grand Slam, that are considered the most renowned. The big four that compose the Grand Slam: Western States 100, Vermont 100, Leadville Trail 100, and Wasatch Front 100. If you complete all of these events in a year, as many ultra-marathoners aspire to, you would log 400 total miles!

The other type is a fixed time period event. The parameter is given: twenty-four hours, forty-eight hours, and six days. The runner who runs the most miles within that time wins. There are also point-to-point events.

Ultimately, there really are no rules in ultra-running. You can stop to eat, rest, walk, and even sleep. It's fairly free and easy. The only penalty for doing these things is that you are losing time doing these things while your competitors are running. How much time are you willing to part with?

Training for Ultra-Runs

The training for an ultra-marathon goes way beyond what is described within this book. There are some similarities and there are some differences. What does not change is that you cannot jump from here to there. Many of the same running principles apply. Building mileage slowly and systematically is a major key to both preparing properly while reducing the likelihood of injury. Stretching is still important.

Physical Preparation

How do many ultra-runners cover these long distances both in practice and during their actual events? The evolution of Jeff Galloway's famous walk/run marathon training program can perhaps be traced to the cornerstone of ultra-training—frequent walking breaks interspersed with running.

The specific ratio of walking to running varies depending to a large degree upon the experience and ability level of the ultra-runner. Some may throw in a two-minute walking break for every mile run. Others may find that walking three minutes for every ten minutes enables them to cover longer and longer distances.

The key point to keep in mind is that walking breaks must be implemented at the beginning of the run or race for this strategy to be effective, not when one's leg muscles are at the point of fatigue or breakdown. In short, regularly scheduled walking breaks greatly increase the ultra-runner's range as opposed to if he or she were to run the entire training or racing distance. Including frequent walking also reduces the wear and tear on the leg muscles, a critical injury prevention strategy.

More competitive ultra-runners will integrate advanced training techniques into their training schedules that emphasize strength and endurance. These will include speed workouts focusing on longer repeat interval distances (800 meters and longer of fast-paced efforts) as well as the inclusion of hill training. In short, their workouts are quite different from those racing much shorter distances, such as the 5K or 10K, although they follow the same advanced training guidelines and precautions. However, ultra-runners practice speedwork and hill training just as was discussed earlier. Nutrition is still paramount. Weight training is still important. And coaches in the sport still caution their runners not to overtrain, if that can sound possible preparing for such an event.

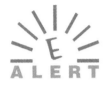

ALERT

Psychologically, the ultra-marathon requires new adjustments. One of the challenges is finding ways to pass hours and hours of time mentally. Ultra-runners comment that there is no limit to the variety of topics they think about while running, ranging from the practical and conventional to the absurd!

Other Preparations

Nutritionally, ultra-marathoners eat greater quantities and more frequently during their events than marathoners. Their training schedules tend to be made up of more long runs than marathoners. Because the weather conditions in these extra-long events can change rapidly (in part due to topographical variations of the course along with the fact that they will often be running morning, noon, and night), ultra-runners must be prepared to add or strip multiple layers of clothing at a moment's notice. The same can be said about terrain. One minute these athletes may be running through the desert, and an hour later they may be climbing a mountain. An ultra-runner has to be thoroughly prepared for the event in which he or she competes.

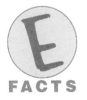

FACTS

Kevin Sayers, the ultra-marathon webmaster and ultra-runner, has completed twenty-seven ultra-marathoning events. He logged 480 miles in events in the year 2000 alone. He ran 300 miles in 1999. And he finished with 590 in 1998! And those are just the races!

Where to Find Out More

After you have run two or three marathons, and you feel like you'd like to attempt an ultra-marathon, it is suggested that you do as much research as possible before going to this next step. Read the Web sites and the magazines, gather information, and look for advice. Whether it be through the advice of a coach or just another experienced ultra-runner, you should try to find someone who can competently guide you to this next level. To put it mildly, the world of ultra-running is not for everybody. It indeed has a limited and select group, though it is gaining in popularity. Exercise caution and prudence when attempting something of this magnitude.

Because ultra-running is still evolving, things change a lot. Thank goodness for the Internet, which can keep up with the frequent changes. Some of the best information repositories for the most current information are on the Web. One of the best ultra-marathon Web sites is *www.fred.net/ultrunr.* This site, Kevin Sayers's Ultra Running Resource (UltRunR) Site, is possibly the best single ultra-runner's site for practical knowledge and training schedules. Everything is covered and the content is provided by a wide range of well-known and experienced ultra-runners. Included within are resources and advice, as well as race schedules and valuable links. Everything is right there.

Likewise, David Blaikie's Ultramarathon World is one of the most up-to-date ultra-running Web sites around (*http://fox.nstn.ca/~dblaikie*). David is a wonderful writer and provides a bird's-eye view for all the events. The site is a veritable who's who of profiles and advice.

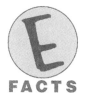

FACTS

There are two magazines that are ultra-running's standard bearers. They are *Marathon & Beyond* (*www.americanultra.org*) and *Ultrarunning* magazine (*www.ultrarunning.com*). They feature high-profile names and interesting articles, as well as calendars.

Ultra-Running Clubs

There are a great many ultra-running clubs around the United States. Contact the AUA or the IAU to find the club nearest you. One of the best links for club information is David Blaikie's Web page. It contains many of the clubs you'll be looking for.

CHAPTER 19

Girls (Women!) Just Want to Have Fun

We all know the adage that men and women are different. Men prefer diners; women like cafés. Men love football; women love Ally McBeal. In the world of running, women and men differ as well. Do women require an entire section unto themselves? In short, yes!

Comparing Men and Women Runners

There are many similarities between men and women runners. Firstly, the biomechanics of running do not differ between men and women. Their posture and arm stride affect their results in the same way. Neither do the training techniques vary from men to women. Both men and women can and should follow the various schedules that have been provided. With little or no variation, both can do the speed workouts, cross-training, weight-training, and stretching that have been discussed earlier in this book. Additionally, men and women routinely run in the same races.

In any of this, little separates the two sexes. However, there are also a great many things that are unique to the female runner. Let's cover a few of the differences here.

Body Type

Contrary to stereotypes, women runners tend to carry more body fat than men—approximately 5 to 10 percent more. Body fat is dead weight, and women need to exert more energy to carry that weight, which saps their strength and stamina. Men tend to have larger hearts and lungs, which allows them to deliver oxygenated blood faster and in greater quantity than their female counterparts. This allows muscles to respond better and faster. Men also tend to have greater muscle mass and stronger bones.

This is not to say that there aren't women runners who don't finish in front of men in a lot of races. However, that is why elite male runners are almost always faster than accomplished women of track and field. This is particularly true in sprinting. However, the gap in performance between elite-caliber men and women narrows as race distances become longer. This is particularly true for race distances of the marathon and beyond.

Menstruation

Certainly the discomforts of menstruation are nothing new to women. However, it must be said that the side effects (bloating, cramps, mood swings) of menstruation can affect their overall participation and performance in both training and racing. At certain times, heavy flow or severe cramps may keep some women from exercising at all.

While the idea of strapping on a pair of running shoes and shorts and hitting the pavement may not seem appealing during menstruation, it's important to remember that exercise at such a time is an excellent idea. The act of sweating alone is an excellent antidote to bloating, which is part of water retention.

Many women runners who exercise regularly have found that they suffer less severe cramps and other monthly discomforts and are, in general, less affected by their menstrual period than women who do not exercise. To the other extreme, there are women who no longer menstruate regularly or at all because they overdo it both in training and racing. While this might not seem like such a bad thing for some women, infrequent or irregular menstrual cycles can lead to an early onset of osteoporosis and interfere with childbearing. It is strongly recommended that women runners discuss their running habits and their monthly menstrual cycle with their doctor from time to time to make sure that they are neither overdoing it nor neglecting important health issues and concerns.

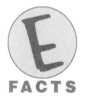

FACTS

Menstruation need not interfere with your competitive urges. Many women runners report little to no change in racing results when they have run competitively during their menstruation period. While they may have run with discomfort, mentally or physically, running seemed to make them feel better in the end.

Fitness for Prenatal Women

Exercise can be part of having a healthy pregnancy. Assuming that it is safe to do so (there are no complications), a woman should try to exercise throughout the duration of pregnancy. Some studies suggest that full benefits are not realized if women stop exercising part of the way through the pregnancy. Of course, if your doctor recommends that you stop exercising due to concerns about your health or the health of the baby, then by all means stop.

FACTS

According to the American College of Obstetricians and Gynecologists (ACOG), "Regular exercise improves a pregnant woman's physical and mental health. Exercising and being fit help a woman during pregnancy and may improve her ability to cope with the pain of labor. Exercise will also make it easier for a woman to get back in shape after the baby is born."

Running Versus Walking

It is important to discuss with your doctor his or her feelings on jogging, running, or walking while you're pregnant. The ability to run well into the second trimester (different women's bodies respond differently to the same athletic stresses) is a decision you must make with your doctor. Many doctors will not insist you give up exercise, but might warn you to either reduce the intensity of or even stop running. Many find walking a very good substitute. It is very important that you and your doctor make this decision together. Many women are loath to give up running until the weight slows them down. Don't press yourself in this situation. Walking is an excellent substitute.

Now that more prenatal (before the birth) and postnatal (after the birth) women are exercising, more continues to be learned about the effects of exercise. In 1994, the ACOG revised its guidelines for exercise during pregnancy and postpartum. One prior guideline that has been dropped concerned exercising at a limited heart rate. The guideline has been revised to reflect the more important issue of women exercising at a level that feels moderate and comfortable.

For most women, exercise during pregnancy is safe and recommended, but in some cases, it is not. If the doctor gives the go-ahead to start a fitness program, a woman should monitor herself during exercise for any changes that may be warning signs of a problem. If any unforeseen concerns or health issues surface, she should immediately contact her doctor for further guidance.

Taking a Prenatal Exercise Class

For some women, taking part in a supervised exercise class can provide assurance and support. Before enrolling in any prenatal program, find out whether the program meets the following criteria:

- The instructor has a fitness or health-related degree and experience or training in obstetrics.
- The instructor is competent to answer fitness- and pregnancy-related questions.
- The instructor incorporates ACOG guidelines and knows warning signs and symptoms with regard to pregnancy.
- A health history and physician's consent are required before joining the class.
- There is an established procedure for management of injuries or emergencies.
- The facility is appropriate for prenatal exercise—it has a supportive floor, mats, and nearby rest rooms, and the exercise room is kept cool.
- The safety and comfort of the participants are never sacrificed.
- The class accommodates varying levels of fitness.
- The class provides frequent breaks to check level of exertion and to hydrate.
- The class includes a warm-up, aerobic exercise, strength and flexibility exercises, and a cool-down.
- The class includes pregnancy-specific needs such as lower back flexibility and pelvic floor exercises.

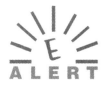

Catherine Cram, an exercise physiologist who specializes in prenatal and postnatal fitness, offers the following advice for a safe and effective prenatal exercise program: Reassess your fitness goals, listen to your body, and consider a supervised prenatal exercise class with a qualified instructor.

Shoes and Clothing

Wear shoes that are one-half to one size larger to allow room for foot swelling. Shoes with Velcro closures can make frequent adjustments easier. Clothing should be comfortable. If overheating is a problem, wear clothing that is nonconstricting, breathes, and wicks moisture away from the body to help stay cool. A sports bra with wide shoulder straps can provide good support, help protect the breasts, and ease or prevent shoulder discomfort.

Forget About Calories

A woman should never exercise to lose weight while pregnant and should not restrict calories for the purpose of preventing weight gain. Mother and fetus need an extra 300 calories a day (for multiple-birth pregnancies, add 300 calories per fetus). To determine whether a woman is eating enough, she should monitor her body weight regularly.

Prenatal women can expect to gain twenty-five to thirty-five pounds. Lean, athletic women who had low levels of body fat before pregnancy may need to gain more. Women who fall into this category may take comfort in knowing that they will recover quickly. If a pregnant woman is not gaining weight (or is losing weight), she needs to increase her caloric intake of nutrient-rich foods. Pregnancy may not be an athletic event, but it is very physically demanding. It is important to remember that the new life presently residing inside the womb needs nutrients and calories to grow and be healthy.

Fitness for Postnatal Women

During the postnatal (or postpartum) period, a woman's body works hard to return to its condition prior to pregnancy. This process can take nearly as long as the pregnancy itself, so be patient. Muscles and skin that stretched to allow for the baby's growth take time to return to their original tone and can make fitting into your old wardrobe challenging. Although this can be emotionally discouraging, it is normal.

FACTS

The following are some prenatal and postnatal fitness guidelines:

- Frequency: Exercise three to five times per week.
- Intensity: Exercise at a level that feels "somewhat hard" to "hard."
- Time: Those just starting an exercise program should only do an aerobic activity five to ten minutes at a time. Those who were fit prior to pregnancy can exercise for twenty to forty-five minutes.

Get Your Doctor's Approval

As in the prenatal stage, a woman in the postnatal period should get approval from her doctor or health care provider before engaging in exercise. If approval is given, the prenatal and postnatal fitness guidelines can be followed until the postnatal period is over (six to twelve months).

The new mother's postnatal condition will affect the timeline of when she can begin as well as what kind of exercise she can start doing. Aside from the physiological adjustments, one of the biggest challenges to a new mother's fitness is finding the availability of free time to work out. But with a little planning, a new mother can carve out a piece of her busy day for exercise that will enhance her physical and emotional health.

Finding Time to Exercise

Couples can designate certain times of the day as "Mom's time" or "Dad's time," when one of them takes care of the baby exclusively (this is outside of the time that either or both of them are at work). This can be a satisfying arrangement for everyone since it allows for each spouse to have some personal time that is exclusively their own.

A rotational schedule can work nicely for grandparents, aunts, uncles, and older siblings to spend time caring for and playing with the baby. Be considerate of others by scheduling a start and a finish time.

Friends, especially those with young children, can fill and share the need to watch the baby while the mother exercises. Again, schedule the time as you would a class or an appointment. Designating a start and a finish time will help you to recruit others; it communicates a respect and appreciation for their time.

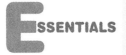

SSENTIALS

Exercise is at least as important as going out for the evening for new mothers. Make an appointment with yourself and arrange a baby-sitter for regular days and times. Unless the mother is training for a marathon, as little as an hour of time can make a huge difference.

Baby-Friendly Equipment

Today's baby-friendly equipment makes it possible for baby to safely go along for Mom's and Dad's walks, jogs, runs, or bike rides. The baby jogger/runner is more stable and durable than a conventional stroller. For bicycling, there are numerous options for baby and child apparatus. There are screened-in trailers, child seats, and mount-on tandem attachments. For safety's sake, be sure that both you and your child wear helmets

Osteoporosis

Osteoporosis is a disease that affects a great many women. Osteoporosis causes bones to be brittle, which can mean the unfortunate end to one's running career. The jarring action of running or a quick fall may cause a fracture or break. Since bone mass often begins to decline after the age of thirty-five or so, that is when women become vulnerable to osteoporosis. The process, if undetected, may accelerate after menopause. However, younger women who have less iron and calcium in their diets, and place too much stress on their bodies, may also contract this disease.

Osteoporosis cannot be reversed. If an affected woman can detect osteoporosis early enough, she can do things, with the help of her doctor, to slow down the disease's progress. A calcium-rich diet is one of the great ways to retard osteoporosis. Running is another. Even though running places stress on bones, it acts as an agent to build stronger bones by automatically reacting to the stress and attempting to increase bone density in the areas where it's greatest. Women runners should discuss osteoporosis with their doctor at their next medical appointment.

Menopause

Menopause is a difficult time for some women and not as difficult for others. Although it may involve deep mood swings, hot flashes, and other discomforts, it need not discourage women from running. There has been no conclusive evidence that running or any other kind of exercise increases or decreases the main effects of menopause. However, there is little doubt that exercise can be a wonderful antidote to stress, depression, anxiety, and a host of other less desirable emotions.

Since menopause can sometimes take as long as ten years to complete its cycle, many women lose their desire and motivation to continue running. Menopause may set in as early as age forty, and most women have passed through menopause by age sixty.

Regardless, there are also many women who are dedicated to their running, and have continued right through their entire menopause, never losing the enjoyment and richness that running brings to their lives. Again, consulting with a physician is the best way to improve your chances of continuing to enjoy running through menopause without physical or mental discomfort or pain.

Safety Tips for Women Runners

While we like to think that we live in a more enlightened time when women are safe running by themselves, it's always a good idea to be aware of potentially unpleasant or dangerous situations. Here are some commonsense suggestions that will help keep you safe.

Don't run in isolated areas, particularly after dark. Whenever possible, run with other people after dark. Vary your running routine. Don't run the same place, the same time, the same day. Mix it up so that strangers can't anticipate when and where you run. Tell a family member, roommate, or friend what your route is and approximately what time you expect to return. Bring a whistle, panic button device, or some other way to attract attention should something happen. Finally, if possible, learn self-defense tactics.

CHAPTER 20

Running Away from Home

N o, this chapter isn't about bailing out on your life and starting all over again! It's about taking your sport with you wherever you go. Remember, the great thing about running is that you really only need your shorts, shirt, and shoes to make it happen. So when you're planning a trip for business or pleasure, don't forget to pack your running gear.

Packing Your Running Gear

Here's how to pack your gear: Designate two small bags to be those to carry your running gear in. One will be for your running shoes (a plastic shopping bag is great for this), and the other will be for your running clothes and necessary accessories. In this bag you'll put your warm-weather gear (shorts, short-sleeved T-shirt or singlet, running bra, etc.) or your cold-weather gear (leggings, thermal top, running bra, long-sleeved T-shirt, gloves, hat, etc.), as well as your all-important running watch. Even if you're going someplace cold and need extra gear, your stuff won't weigh much. Wouldn't you rather lug around the extra pounds your gear weighs than the extra pounds you'll weigh if you don't run while you're gone?

But It's a Vacation!

True, vacations are times when you leave the stresses and worries of your daily routine behind and indulge in the good life. For a lot of us, that means rest and relaxation with fun stuff like sightseeing, dining out, dancing, reading, sunbathing, and other leisure activities thrown in. Do you see running on this list? No. Would most of your friends call you crazy if you told them you were looking forward to getting your five miles a day in on your trip to the Grand Canyon? Probably, but remember, it's your time off, not theirs!

Reasons to Run on Vacation

Think of it this way. If you've got a running routine set up because you wanted to get in shape and lose weight, you're probably already seeing results and maybe you're actually starting to enjoy running itself! When you go on vacation and indulge in big meals, drinks, and extra sleep, those pounds and inches are going to come back in no time—unless, of course, you can get in a few runs. Even short runs will keep your metabolism humming and ensure you don't regress. You'll enjoy that piña colada even more knowing you earned it by getting in some aerobic exercise.

If you're in training for a half-marathon or marathon, or even if you've recently completed one, not getting your miles in for a couple of weeks could throw you off. You don't want to undermine all the hard work and miles you've put in before your trip by not keeping up with your running during the trip.

FACTS

There are very few places on earth where you can't get a run in. You need the proper equipment, of course, but after that, it's a matter of motivation. Would you like to get a run in before the big business dinner you need to attend? Runs on the road are great ways to stay in shape and stay focused and refreshed.

Vacation Running and Romance

Perhaps you and your significant other lead busy lives and you're going away to rekindle the romance in your relationship. However, your significant other is not a runner and you don't want to take away from your time together. Just remind him or her (and yourself) that regular exercise helps you feel better and look better. It improves your circulation, your overall good health, your energy level, your mental acuity, and your appetite. Wouldn't Dr. Ruth call these ingredients important for a healthy sex life? You bet she would! In fact, perhaps you and your significant other can begin participating in sports or exercise together while you're away. It's a great way to bond and have fun.

ESSENTIALS

Which sounds better to you: Wining and dining under the stars until you're tired and stuffed, or getting in a twenty- to thirty-minute run with your partner, having a big glass of water, and emerging refreshed from a hot shower?

Run to See the Sights

Besides the very important and very real benefits of maintaining your training and fitness goals while you're on the road, many runners agree the greatest satisfaction of running away from home is exploring new places. Let's face it, there's nothing like running through a new neighborhood to reinvigorate your runs. It's fun to see how people in other parts of the country and the world decorate their homes and their yards, configure their streets, go about their daily lives.

If you're traveling in a rural area, your runs may take you past apple orchards you wouldn't have otherwise found, through forests your spouse or kids wouldn't be interested in but you find beautiful, up hills that are more challenging than those you're used to, along coastlines that tourists typically avoid—the possibilities are endless. Not only are you getting your exercise in, but you're getting an up-close-and-personal look at a new part of the world. You'll be amazed at how invigorating this is.

Don't be surprised if you start remembering your trips by the runs you took instead of the meals you ate, the museums you visited, the theme park you spent a month's salary at, even the family stories you heard for the first time. When you're on your run, the time is yours. Even if it's a quick twenty minutes, being out there on your own in a new place will revive all your senses.

ESSENTIALS

If you've gotten into the very good habit of keeping a running log or journal, it will come in especially handy when you're traveling. Take notes about the things you liked best about your run and the things you liked least. In this way, your running log becomes your travel journal.

Planning for Safety

If fitness and adventure are one part of the equation of going running while away from home, safety is the other. Because as exciting as it is to be in new places, the truth is it's not familiar territory for you. Taking a wrong turn somewhere could get you lost easier than you think. If you don't speak the language, have no map with you, or it starts getting dark, you could be in big trouble. And while most runners would agree it's particularly gratifying to do some of these runs alone, running by yourself exposes you to more dangers—anything from twisting your ankle while running a trail to accidentally running into the "bad" part of town.

Use Common Sense

These frightening scenarios are easily avoided by following commonsense safety rules. First, trust your instincts. If a business trip on a limited budget puts you in a hotel where there's nothing but strip malls and highways everywhere you look, you may have to either use the hotel gym or limit your run to laps around the parking lot. You certainly don't want to be running anywhere near a busy street or highway where cars are making quick turns or going at high speeds, not to mention your vulnerability in a setting like this. Strip malls are notorious for spontaneous drag racing or "cruising," multiple intersections, and lots of visual distractions, all of which make it that much harder for drivers to see you out there running.

Likewise, if you're a bit behind schedule and you get to your hotel, campsite or bed and breakfast at dusk instead of earlier in the afternoon, however beautiful it may appear, you should consider postponing your run until morning when you have the full advantage of daylight. Once you know a trail or an area and have gauged how far or long it is to run it, then you may want to consider running at dusk. But don't run anywhere new in the dark. Even if for some reason you've done it before, don't let your cocky side make this decision for you. You were tempting fate if you did it once. Don't do it again.

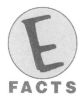

FACTS

There are certain areas in life where risk-taking can pay off big time. Running on the road is not one of them. If you wouldn't want a member of your family or one of your best friends to go out on the run you're considering, then don't do it yourself.

Another commonsense safety rule is to leave a message with somebody about the fact that you're going for a run. If you're traveling by yourself, you should leave a note in your hotel room, tent, or wherever you're staying. Indicate the time you left and how long you expect to be out.

Another easy and practical thing to do is ask at the front desk if there's a running trail that's accessible from the hotel. The staff is usually happy to tell you all about it, and they'll tell you if there are loops of different lengths in case you want to do three miles one day and ten another, for example. After getting the lowdown from the staff, you can let them know that you're going out on that trail and you expect it to take you a half hour, for example. Leave your name and your room number with the hotel personnel.

When you get back, if the staff you spoke with are still at the desk, you can tell them what you thought about the trail and thank them for their help. This will encourage them to share the information with other hotel guests who are looking for a nice run.

If you're traveling with others, make sure they know to expect you back within a certain time. Be generous with the time, but not overly so. You don't want them calling the police if you're not back in forty-five minutes like you said because you decided you wanted to go just a bit farther. On the other hand, you don't want them to figure you're just out enjoying yourself if you're not back within a few hours.

While on the run, carry identification with you. Write your name, home address and phone number and the name, address, and phone number of the place you're staying on a piece of paper that you can fold up and hold in your hand or tuck into a pocket or gear holder. Don't wear anything that could make you a target, such as sparkly jewelry, your most expensive wristwatch, etc.

ALERT

When running in a new place, you may need a fanny pack or a wrist or ankle attachment that can hold a few small things like your hotel key, a few dollars in pocket change, and certainly identification. Look in running stores or online suppliers for these kinds of things and then go for a practice run. You'll need to feel comfortable but not conspicuous.

You must wear or carry a timepiece with you. The best thing, of course, is your waterproof, lightweight stopwatch or training watch that you bought along with your other necessary gear for running. But if you forgot it, wear or carry your regular watch. Since you'll be setting off into the unknown, time is your best bearing.

When you run, figure you want to go fifteen or twenty minutes out, then fifteen or twenty minutes back. Just as when you drive someplace new then go back, getting there can seem to take longer than the return journey. That's because your senses are working overtime to catch everything new. The same thing will happen on your run. You'll be busy looking around and taking it all in. Keep an eye on your watch. It'll seem like you've been out longer than your watch says; but when you get to the time that is your halfway turnaround time and you start to head back, you'll enjoy reliving the sights from the run out and time will go by more quickly.

More Safety Tips

There's an excellent Web site called Run the Planet (*www.runtheplanet.com*) that's loaded with tips and advice on where and when to run around the world. On the site is a section called "Safety on the Run," by the Hudson Mohawk Road Runners Club. Besides the tips already offered in this chapter, here are some especially good ones from their page:

- Be alert at all times and be wary of "runner's high," fatigue, or any lapse of concentration.
- Use your ears as well as your eyes—don't wear headphones.
- Avoid running when relative humidity exceeds 90 percent.
- Consider another form of exercise when adverse weather conditions make running dangerous.
- Know where police are usually to be found and where businesses, stores, offices are likely to be open and active.
- When in doubt, follow your intuition and avoid potential trouble; if something seems suspicious, do not panic, but run in a different direction.
- If the same car cruises past you more than once, take down even a partial license number and make it obvious that you are aware of its presence (but keep your distance).
- If confronted, ignore jeers and verbal harassment, and keep moving.
- Rather than approaching a car to give directions or the time of day, point toward the nearest police or information source, shrug your shoulders, and keep moving.

Run the Planet also has travel safety links posted on its site. These include Embassy World, a listing of all the embassies and consulates around the world; foreign entry requirements for U.S. citizens traveling on business or pleasure; a site that defines what certain body gestures mean in countries around the world (you'd be surprised!); the International Society of Travel Medicine; and travel warnings from various consulates.

Hooking Up with Other Runners

Depending on the type of travel you're doing, it may be easy for you to hook up with other runners—or not. If you're on a business trip with associates who you know also run, you can ask them if they want to meet for a group run. If you're at a large hotel or convention center, you can ask the staff of the health club if they know any other runners who are guests at the hotel who might want to run with someone. Or you might just see someone else in the lobby when you're coming down for your run. Think about going together!

Just don't shed your common sense in your enthusiasm to explore and exercise. If the hotel hooks you up with someone who doesn't seem like your type, make up an excuse to get out of the run. It's your personal time, and you are not obligated to run with someone even if the hotel did the work to find a running partner for you. Likewise, don't be offended if this other person seems to lose interest in running with you. No big deal, just go enjoy your run.

One thing that's true no matter where you run is that no one gets too offended if you decide to change your mind. So if you or the person you were supposed to run with don't hit it off for some reason, just say, "Thanks for meeting me here," and "See you later. Have a nice run."

Running with Business Associates

Remember, too, that if you're on a business trip, you might end up jogging alongside the CEO—or a new assistant. In the same way that it's unprofessional to drink too much at a company function and start gossiping or sharing information that may not be appropriate for the other person to hear, the same holds true for informal meetings like runs. If the CEO wants your opinion about the department you work in, even if you're miserable, find something positive to say, at least to start the conversation. If he or she prods you, be tactful. You want to leave a senior manager with the impression that you're a team player and a smart person, someone who understands where the company's going and has constructive ideas about how to contribute.

If you don't have ideas, here's your opportunity to see if the CEO will share some of his or her vision with you! Ask what his or her favorite aspects are of the job, or ask about how their prior experience is influencing their current position. Most people love to talk about themselves.

You want to leave a junior-level employee with a good impression, too. Remember, this level of employee is the one who's got his or her ear to the pipeline. If they go back to their peer group and say, *Hey, Mr. Jones in accounting has been here five years and he says the company is on the verge of some great new growth*, you know that news will spread fast!

When you're sharing a positive activity that makes you feel good, it's easy to feel an instant camaraderie. In a business setting, however, don't mistake camaraderie for a window to "tell all." You don't have to talk about business at all, if you don't want to. Instead, talk about where you run at home, races you've run, or how long you've been running.

Racing on the Road

Another great way to get an invigorating workout while on a business or pleasure trip is to enter a local race. Go online a few weeks before you're scheduled to leave and do a search for local running clubs in the area you're planning to visit. Go to their Web sites and see what's on the race calendar. Call the contact person for the race to get more information on the size of the event, whether it's a hilly or flat course, if there's a post-race party or fair, and so on. If you decide to do the race, ask for directions from the place you'll be staying to the race and ask how long it should take to get there.

FACTS

Many cities have special races to celebrate holidays like Thanksgiving, Halloween, Memorial Day, Labor Day, and New Year's. New York City's Midnight Run on New Year's Eve draws thousands of runners from all over the world to run a 5K through Central Park at midnight, accompanied by fireworks and non-alcoholic champagne. It's an extremely festive and fun way to start a new year.

Marathoning Around the World

Why not do a really big race in a new place? That's what legions of marathoners from around the world choose to do. Often you can get a good rate to travel and stay someplace for a week, you're traveling with like-minded folks, you don't have to worry too much about how much you eat while you're there (though of course you want to avoid foods that are too exotic, especially before the race), and you have an instant sightseeing tour. Marathoning in foreign places is a way of making the race the focus of the vacation. The race chooses you and you go to it to see what it's all about.

It's easy to find information on running marathons in all corners of the world. Start at *www.runnersworld.com* or buy the *Runner's World* magazine, and you'll be on your way.

The Dublin and Paris Marathons

Irish Americans love to run the Dublin Marathon. In this "fair city," so the song goes, Sweet Molly Malone wheeled her wheelbarrow through streets broad and narrow. It's going to take a livelier tune to sustain you through 26.2 in Ireland's capital, but you probably won't have time to hum it since there's lots to look at and listen to along the course.

For Francophiles, the Paris Marathon is *magnifique!* What better way to see the City of Lights than by running through the *arrondissements*, ogling the bread and cheese. Dinner will be wonderful the night after the marathon!

Favorite Running Cities

The folks at *Runner's World*, ever on the go, decided to rate the ten best running cities in the United States. How did they do it? According to them, they "gathered everyone on staff and came up with a laundry list: great trails, great weather, little pollution, little traffic, low crime, lots of races, and lots of running clubs." They got feedback from runners who both live in those cities and who run on their travels, and they polled their top columnists/runners, like Jeff Galloway and Hal Higdon. Here's their list of Top Ten:

- Boulder, Colorado
- Minneapolis and St. Paul, Minnesota
- Colorado Springs, Colorado
- Sacramento, California
- Jacksonville, Florida
- Eugene, Oregon
- Atlanta, Georgia
- San Luis Obispo, California
- Boston, Massachusetts
- Tampa, Florida

If you go online to *www.runnersworld.com* and look up the article "10 Best Running Cities" by Bill Donohue, you can get a description of each city's best running features and a number of Web sites that give you more information on the city itself or races being held there.

New York, New York

Nothing beats running in Central Park, an oasis in the biggest and most exciting city in the world. Strap on your running shoes and prepare to be wowed. You'll join thousands of runners on their daily loops through Central Park, becoming one with fellow exercisers on roller blades and bicycles, passing horse-drawn carriages, and seeing strollers of every nationality. You'll pass the restaurant Tavern on the Green and the Metropolitan Museum of Art.

Head uptown to the Reservoir where joggers have a 1.5-mile trail practically all to themselves with some of the best views of the skyline you can find. The New York City Road Runners Club sponsors races almost every weekend, including fun ones like the April Fool's Backward Mile. There's no better way to feel connected to this imposing city as a traveler than to participate in the ritual of running with the natives in their inner-city playground.

Chicago, Illinois

From wherever you're staying in Chicago, it's not far to Lake Shore Drive, which runs along the shores of Lake Michigan. Yes, the Drive is a roadway, but there's a walking/running path that parallels it. Talk about some nice skyline views! You'll get a great perspective on the Windy City as you run past Soldier Field, the aquarium, the art museum, the pier, and down to the more residential part of town. Depending on the time of year, be prepared for anything from humidity to arctic air. One thing's for sure, you'll get that breeze off the lake to aid or challenge you. What better way to gear up for a night of blues music and barbeque than to get in a run before dinner?

Waterbury, Vermont

With the world-class ski resorts of Stowe and Sugarbush close by, Waterbury is also an almost picture-perfect Vermont town of church spires, antique shops, and quaint village streets. And then there are the foothills of the Green Mountains. You can't run in Waterbury without going up them—and down them. But your legs won't mind when your senses are filled with the beauty of Vermont on a fall day, or blanketed in new snow, or turning green in spring. Even summer provides a visual feast of mottled sun and shade ripe with the scent of pine. If you're not used to running hills, though, take it easy going up and down. An old saying says going down is for your legs, going up is for your heart. Take it easy on both and don't overexert yourself. Enjoy the challenge.

Washington, D.C.

One of the country's most popular marathons is the Marine Corps Marathon, called both "The People's Marathon" and "The Monuments Marathon." Why? Because the 26.2-mile course snakes through our nation's capital's monuments, including the Capitol, the Pentagon, the Smithsonian Institution, the Kennedy Center, and the Lincoln, Jefferson, and Washington Monuments. It's a race and a history lesson all in one. As a business or leisure traveler, you don't have to do the whole marathon course to experience the beauty and history in and around this city. And the areas just adjacent to D.C., such as Arlington, Virginia, and Georgetown, are also beautiful for running and touring.

Charleston, South Carolina

Charleston was first settled in 1670, ranking it as one of this country's oldest and most historic cities. The area is quite diverse culturally, recreationally, and geographically with so much to see and do. From it's beautiful beaches, parks, antebellum plantations, tidal creeks and marshes, and of course, its beautiful downtown historic district, you will want to spend, at a minimum, three days to even begin to experience Charleston's charm and beauty. There's no shortage of lodging and restaurants; Charleston ranks just second behind New York City in the number of restaurants per capita.

Without question, the best way to tour Charleston is not by one of those famous carriage tours, but rather by foot. Stay downtown for a few extra bucks or park at Colonial Lake, the City Marina, the Battery, Waterfront Park, or the South Carolina Aquarium to begin your run or walk. Meandering through the historic district or running along the waterfront is like traveling back in time as you'll see dozens upon dozens of well-preserved, maintained, and fully functional commercial and residential buildings that date back to the late 1700s and 1800s. Take a close look and you will see beautifully manicured gardens, quaint courtyards, piazzas (Charleston's term for porches), wrought iron gates, exquisitely crafted doors, and more.

There are a host of other options for touring the area on the run, too many to adequately cover in a couple of paragraphs. The pedestrian sidewalks on several of Charleston's bridges offer spectacular vantage points for views of the Charleston peninsula, harbor, Ashley and Cooper Rivers, marshes, and more. Two of these include the James Island Connector and Cooper River Bridge. The later is the central attraction for the 25,000 plus participants who run/walk this famous springtime 10K race that bears its name. Drive to Charles Towne Landing State Park, the site where Charles Towne was first settled, and run among the beautiful oak trees. Other recreational sites that offer paths on which to take in beautiful sights include Hampton Park as well as James Island, Palmetto Islands, and Wannamaker County Parks. Drive to any of the three area barrier islands (Folly Beach, Sullivan's Island, or Isle of Palms) and run on the beach or through the neighborhoods in these communities.

ESSENTIALS   Whether your travels take you to one of these top-rated running cities or not, you're guaranteed great memories of all your travels if you follow the advice in this chapter and run away from home. It's addicting!

APPENDIX A

Finding a Running Club, at Home or Abroad

Search Engines

There are a great number of excellent running clubs around the world that are easy to find, inexpensive to join, and which sponsor activities that you can participate in for either a particular weekend or all year. Many of the best-known running clubs are those associated with well-known marathons, such as the Boston Athletic Club, the New York Road Runners Club, and so forth. One of the best ways to locate a running club near you is to search some of the sites that follow.

If you want to see what the World Wide Web brings you via search engines like Yahoo! and Google, go to those sites and search for "running clubs." Or type in "Running Clubs and Teams." More than 200 running Web sites will come up. Even this is not complete, but it's an excellent start. Or, you can scroll down the endless list of Web site matches, hoping to find one close to you. As with most searches, you're bound to find a lot of sites of interest even beyond what you were originally looking for.

The United States

In the United States, the best place to start is with the granddaddy of them all: The Road Runners Club of America (RRCA). Not only can you find local and national clubs through the RRCA, you can get an idea of what's happening in running across the country. To find clubs in the state where you live, or a state you're planning to visit, you can go straight to a map on their Web site, click on the state, and it immediately lists all the running clubs in that state. It's wonderful! The RRCA's contact information is as follows:

> **RRCA National Office**
> 510 North Washington Street
> Alexandria, VA 22314
> email: office@rrca.org
> phone: (703) 836-0558
> fax: (703) 836-4430
> *www.rrca.org*

Canada

Like the United States, Canada has lots of running clubs that offer organized events for their members and guests. Online searches can yield you lots of results, and this list of organizations across the country should help, as well.

Boreal Running Club
Montreal, Quebec
(514) 624-3320

Capital City Road Runners Club
P.O. Box 20104
Fredericton,
New Brunswick E3B 6Y8

Hershey Harriers
Vancouver, B.C.
(604) 682-8094

Kootenay Lake Joggers Club
5746 Upper Long Beach Rd.
RR#3 S-14 C-4
Nelson BC V1L 5P6
(604) 229 5368

Lions Gate Road Runners
3482 Nairn
Vancouver, BC V5S 4B5

Marathon Dynamics Running Club
(416) 250-0552

Mississauga Track and Field Club
3075 Gambin Court
Mississauga On L5A 3Z6

Mississippi Running Club
P.O. Box 285
Carleton Place ON K7C 3P4
(613) 257-7873

Ottawa Athletic Club Racing Team
79A Glenpark Drive
Gloucester, ON K1B 3Z1
(613) 824-0183

Peloton Athletic Club
32-3495 Rue St-Dominique
Montreal, Quebec H2X 2X5
(514) 285-0080

Penticton Pounders
Box 20056
Penticton, BC V2A 8K3

Prairie Inn Harriers Running Club
Victoria, B.C.
(250) 381-IRUN (4786)

Queen's T. & F. Dept. of Athletics
Queen's University
Kingston, ON K7L 3N6

Running Room Running Club LTD
321A-10th St. N.W.
Calgary, AB T2N 1V7
(403) 270-7317

Wapiti Striders Road Running Club
Box 1495
Grande Prairie, AB T8V 4Z3
(403) 532-7138

Stouffville Stompers
10646-63 Avenue
Edmonton, AB T6H 1P6
(403) 435-6583

Whitehorse Athletic Club
44 MacPherson Rd
Whitehorse, Yukon Y1A 5S4
(403) 668-4052

"Turtles" Running and Brunch Club
c/o Riley Park Community Center
50 E. 30th Ave.
Vancouver, BC V5V 2T9
(604) 879-6222

Finding a Running Club Outside of the United States and Canada

Again, thank goodness for the World Wide Web! There's a great site that provides an excellent international directory. It's called the Running Page, and it's at *www.runningpage.com*. Even if participating in an event on another continent isn't in your immediate plans, this site will educate and inspire.

Appendix B

Magazines and Books on Running

Magazines

Don't you love your magazine subscriptions? There in your mailbox, behind all the bills and junk mail, is an escape into a whole different world, whether it's one of news, sports, decorating, gender issues, or a particular hobby. And so it is with a magazine on running. Once you're hooked on the sport, you'll enjoy reading about how other people are fascinated with it, too. Some of the most popular and well-known running magazines are listed below.

Runner's World
Rodale, Inc.
Emmaus, PA 18098
(610) 967-8809
www.runnersworld.com

Running Journal
PO Box 157
Greeneville, TN 37743
(423) 638-4177
www.running.net

Running Research News
R.R.N. P.O. Box 27041
Lansing, MI 48909
(517) 371- 4897
(517) 371-4447 (fax)
www.rrnews.com

Running Times
213 Danbury Road
Wilton, CT 06897
(203) 761-1113
www.runningtimes.com

Marathon & Beyond
411 Park Lane Dr.
Champaign, IL 61820
(217) 359-9345
www.marathonandbeyond.com

Trail Runner
North South Publications
5455 Spine Road, Mezzanine A
Boulder, CO 80301
(303) 499-8410
www.trailrunnermag.com

Ultrarunning
P.O. BOX 890238
Weymouth, MA 02189-0238
(781) 340-0616
www.ultrarunning.com

Track & Field News
2570 El Camino Real, Suite 606
Mountain View, CA 94040
(650) 948-8188
www.trackandfieldnews.com

Books

If you enjoy reading about running, you've already got one of the best books out there—this one! But like all sports and hobbies, running has a deep and wide body of works that make up its library. These may include books on training for particular events, books on health and injuries, books on the psychology of running, and books for the pure enjoyment of running. And of course there are new books coming out all the time. This list is not all-inclusive, but it includes classics like the works of Dr. George Sheehan, Bob Glover, Jeff Galloway, Amby Burfoot, and Joan Benoit Samuelson.

Two publishers that specialize in books on running and physical fitness are Rodale Press in Emmaus, PA, and Human Kinetics Publications in Champaign, IL. Many of their titles are listed below. You can also look up their entire libraries online by going to *www.rodale.com* and *www.humankinetics.com*.

General Training and Inspiration

Battista, Garth, ed. *The Runner's Literary Companion: Great Stories and Poems About Running.* (Penguin USA, 1996)

Bloom, Marc. *Run With the Champions : Training Programs and Secrets of America's 50 Greatest Runners.* (Rodale, 2001)

Burfoot, Amby. *The Principles of Running.* (Rodale, 1999)

Burfoot, Amby. *The Runner's Guide to the Meaning of Life: What 35 Years of Running Has Taught Me About Winning, Losing, Happiness, Humility, and the Human Heart.* (Rodale, 2000)

Burfoot, Amby. *Runner's World Complete Book of Running: Everything You Need to Know to Run for Fun, Fitness, and Competition.* (Rodale, 1999)

Couch, Jean. *The Runner's Yoga Book: A Balanced Approach to Fitness.* (Rodmell Press, 1992)

Daniels, Jack. *Daniels' Running Formula.* (Human Kinetics, 1998)

Ellis, Joe and Joe Henderson. *Running Injury-Free : How to Prevent, Treat, and Recover from Dozens of Painful Problems.* (Rodale, 1994)

Galloway, Jeff. *Galloway's Book on Running.* (Shelter Publications, 1984)

Galloway, Jeff. *Jeff Galloway's Training Journal.* (Phidippides Publication, 1998)

Glover, Bob and Shelly-Lynn Florence Glover. *The Competitive Runner's Handbook: The Bestselling Guide to Running 5Ks Through Marathons.* (Penguin USA, 1999)

Glover, Bob. *The Runner's Handbook: The Best-Selling Classic Fitness Guide for Beginner and Intermediate Runners.* (Penguin USA, 1996)

Glover, Bob and Shelly-Lynn Florence Glover. *The Runner's Training Diary: For Fitness Runners and Competitive Racers.* (Penguin USA, 1997)

Henderson, Joe. *Best Runs.* (Human Kinetics, 1998)

Henderson, Joe and Jeff Galloway. *Better Runs: 25 Years' Worth of Lessons for Running Faster and Farther.* (Human Kinetics, 1995)

Henderson, Joe and Hal Higdon. *Running 101.* (Human Kinetics, 2000)

Higdon, Hal. *Hal Higdon's How to Train: The Best Programs, Workouts, and Schedules for Runners of All Ages.* (Rodale, 1997)

Higdon, Hal. *Hal Higdon's Smart Running: Expert Advice on Training, Motivation, Injury Prevention, Nutrition, and Good Health for Runners of Any Age and Ability.* (Rodale, 1998)

Higdon, Hal. *Run Fast: How to Beat Your Best Time Every Time.* (Rodale, 2000)

Higdon, Hal. *Run Fast: How to Train for a 5K or 10K Race.* (Rodale, 2000)

Lynch, Jerry and Warren A. Scott. *Running Within: A Guide to Mastering the Body-Mind-Spirit Connection for Ultimate Training and Racing.* (Human Kinetics, 1999)

MacNeill, Ian. *Beginning Runner's Handbook: The Proven 13-Week Walk Run Program.* (Greystone Publishing, 1999)

Martin, David E. and Peter N. Coe. *Better Training for Distance Runners.* (Human Kinetics, 1997)

McMillan, Greg and Juliana Risner. *Zap! You're a Runner.* (Road Runner Sports, 1999)

Nelson, Kevin. *The Runner's Book of Daily Inspiration: A Year of Motivation, Revelation, and Instruction.* (McGraw Hill, 1999)

Noakes, Tim. *Lore of Running.* (Human Kinetics, 1991)

Parker, Jr., John L. *Once a Runner.* (Cedarwinds Publishing Company, 1998)

Raythorn, Dennis and Rich Hanna. *The Ultimate Runner's Journal: Your Daily Training Partner and Log.* (Marathon Publishing, 1998)

Reese, Paul. *The Old Man and the Road: Reflections While Completing a Crossing of All 50 States on Foot at Age 80.* (Keokee Co. Publishers, 2000)

Runner's World Magazine. *Runner's World: Training Diary.* (Hungry Minds, annual)

Scott, Dagny and Amby Burfoot. *Runner's World Complete Book of Women's Running: The Best Advice to Get Started, Stay Motivated, Lose Weight, Run Injury-Free, Be Safe, and Train for Any Distance.* (Rodale, 2000)

Sheehan, George. *Dr. George Sheehan on Getting Fit and Feeling Great: How to Feel Great 24 Hours a Day/Running and Being/This Running Life/Three Volumes in One.* (Listen U.S.A., 1985)

Sheehan, George. *George Sheehan on Running to Win: How to Achieve the Physical, Mental & Spiritual Victories of Running.* (Rodale, 1994)

Sheehan, George. *Going the Distance: One Man's Journey to the End of His Life.* (Villard Books, 1996)

Sheehan, George. *Personal Best: The Foremost Philosopher of Fitness Shares Techniques and Tactics for Success and Self-Liberation.* (Rodale, 1992)

Sheehan, George. *Running and Being: The Total Experience.* (Second Wind II Llc, 1998)

Svensson, Sharon L. *The Total Runner's Log: The Essential Training Tool for the Runner.* (Trimarket, 1998)

Weisenfeld, Murray. *The Runner's Repair Manual.* (St. Martin's Press, 1981)

Will-Weber, Mark, ed. *Quotable Runner: Great Moments of Wisdom, Inspiration, Wrongheadedness, and Humor.* (Breakaway Books, 1995)

Marathon Training

Bloch, Gordon Bakoulis. *How to Train for and Run Your Best Marathon.* (Fireside, 1993)

Galloway, Jeff. *Marathon!* (Phidippides Publications, 2000)

Hanc, John and Grete Waitz. *The Essential Marathoner: A Concise Guide to the Race of Your Life.* (Lyons Press, 1996)

Henderson, Joe. *Marathon Training: The Proven 100-Day Program for Success.* (Human Kinetics, 1997)

Higdon, Hal. *Marathon: The Ultimate Training Guide.* (Rodale, 1999)

Kuehls, Dave. *4 Months to a 4-Hour Marathon.* (Perigee, 1998)

Pfitzinger, Pete and Scott Douglas. *Advanced Marathoning.* (Human Kinetics, 2001)

Whitsett, David A. *The Non-Runner's Marathon Trainer.* (McGraw Hill, 1998)

Marathon History

Boeder, Robert B. *Beyond the Marathon: The Grand Slam of Trail Ultrarunning.* (Old Mountain Press, 1996)

Connelly, Michael. *26 Miles to Boston: The Boston Marathon Experience from Hopkinton to Copley Square.* (Parnassus Imprints, 1998)

Derderian, Tom and Joan Benoit Samuelson. *Boston Marathon: The First Century of the World's Premier Running Event.* (Human Kinetics, 1996)

Lovett, Charles C. *The Olympic Marathon: A Centennial History of the Games' Most Storied Race.* (Praeger Publications, 1997)

Martin, David E and Roger W. H. Gynn. *The Olympic Marathon.* (Human Kinetics, 2000)

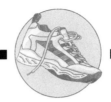

APPENDIX C
Running Online

General Sites

Cool Running—Race calendars, training tips, information on youth running, it's all here. *www.coolrunning.com*

Kick—"The Complete Online Resource for Runners." *www.kicksports.com*

Runners Web—A running and triathlon resource site. *www.runnersweb.com*

Road Runners Club of America—675 clubs and 190,000 members throughout America. *www.rrca.org*

Running Amuck—A huge list of running links. *www.fix.net/~doogie/links.html*

Running Free—A collection of widgets and advice for distance runners. *http://home.connectnet.com/eoinf*

On the Run—Your online source for the long distance running community. *www.ontherun.com*

Running Network—The most comprehensive source of information for grassroots runners online. *www.runningnetwork.com*

Runner's World Magazine—It's not just a Web site for the magazine; it's a world of advice for runners. *www.runnersworld.com*

Running on the Web—A list of running-related sites. *http://sorrel.humboldt.edu/~rrw1/runweb.html*

Dr. Pribut's Sports Medicine Page—A site with lots of helpful sports medicine information. *www.drpribut.com*

Global Health and Fitness—Tells you everything you need to know to eat right, stay in shape, and feel great. *www.global-fitness.com*

Marathon Training Web Sites

State of the Art Marathon Training—Offers a wide range of running topics designed to meet the needs of the beginner to the advanced competitor. *www.marathontraining.com*

Hal Higdon On the Run—Provides advice from a foremost marathon competitor and trainer. *www.halhigdon.com*

Jeff Galloway's Marathon Training Program—Check out the official site for the guy who started a marathoning revolution. *www.jeffgalloway.com*

U.S.A. Fit—"Change your life" with helpful marathon tips. *www.usafit.com*

Association of International Marathons and Road Races—Tap into the international running community here. *www.aims-association.org*

YOU Can Run a Marathon—Offers all kinds of advice to educate and inspire. *www.expage.com/page/marathon*

Ultra-Marathoning

Ultra-Running Resource Site—Gives you information on every aspect of ultra-running. *www.fred.net/ultrunr*

Official Web site of the Western States 100—A great site to look at to understand what's involved in an endurance run. *www.ws100.com*

American Ultra-Running Association—A resource for news and information on ultra-running in the United States. *www.americanultra.org*

Stan "Runs 100s" Jensen—An ultra-runner's personal Web site, full of useful links and information. *www.run100s.com*

Ultrarunning Online—Provides interesting articles and photos for ultra-runners. *www.ultrarunning.com*

Index

We Have EVERYTHING!

Everything® **After College Book**
$12.95, 1-55850-847-3

Everything® **American History Book**
$12.95, 1-58062-531-2

Everything® **Angels Book**
$12.95, 1-58062-398-0

Everything® **Anti-Aging Book**
$12.95, 1-58062-565-7

Everything® **Astrology Book**
$12.95, 1-58062-062-0

Everything® **Baby Names Book**
$12.95, 1-55850-655-1

Everything® **Baby Shower Book**
$12.95, 1-58062-305-0

Everything® **Baby's First Food Book**
$12.95, 1-58062-512-6

Everything® **Baby's First Year Book**
$12.95, 1-58062-581-9

Everything® **Barbeque Cookbook**
$12.95, 1-58062-316-6

Everything® **Bartender's Book**
$9.95, 1-55850-536-9

Everything® **Bedtime Story Book**
$12.95, 1-58062-147-3

Everything® **Bicycle Book**
$12.00, 1-55850-706-X

Everything® **Breastfeeding Book**
$12.95, 1-58062-582-7

Everything® **Build Your Own Home Page**
$12.95, 1-58062-339-5

Everything® **Business Planning Book**
$12.95, 1-58062-491-X

Everything® **Candlemaking Book**
$12.95, 1-58062-623-8

Everything® **Casino Gambling Book**
$12.95, 1-55850-762-0

Everything® **Cat Book**
$12.95, 1-55850-710-8

Everything® **Chocolate Cookbook**
$12.95, 1-58062-405-7

Everything® **Christmas Book**
$15.00, 1-55850-697-7

Everything® **Civil War Book**
$12.95, 1-58062-366-2

Everything® **Classical Mythology Book**
$12.95, 1-58062-653-X

Everything® **Collectibles Book**
$12.95, 1-58062-645-9

Everything® **College Survival Book**
$12.95, 1-55850-720-5

Everything® **Computer Book**
$12.95, 1-58062-401-4

Everything® **Cookbook**
$14.95, 1-58062-400-6

Everything® **Cover Letter Book**
$12.95, 1-58062-312-3

Everything® **Creative Writing Book**
$12.95, 1-58062-647-5

Everything® **Crossword and Puzzle Book**
$12.95, 1-55850-764-7

Everything® **Dating Book**
$12.95, 1-58062-185-6

Everything® **Dessert Book**
$12.95, 1-55850-717-5

Everything® **Digital Photography Book**
$12.95, 1-58062-574-6

Everything® **Dog Book**
$12.95, 1-58062-144-9

Everything® **Dreams Book**
$12.95, 1-55850-806-6

Everything® **Etiquette Book**
$12.95, 1-55850-807-4

Everything® **Fairy Tales Book**
$12.95, 1-58062-546-0

Everything® **Family Tree Book**
$12.95, 1-55850-763-9

Everything® **Feng Shui Book**
$12.95, 1-58062-587-8

Everything® **Fly-Fishing Book**
$12.95, 1-58062-148-1

Everything® **Games Book**
$12.95, 1-55850-643-8

Everything® **Get-A-Job Book**
$12.95, 1-58062-223-2

Everything® **Get Out of Debt Book**
$12.95, 1-58062-588-6

Everything® **Get Published Book**
$12.95, 1-58062-315-8

Everything® **Get Ready for Baby Book**
$12.95, 1-55850-844-9

Everything® **Get Rich Book**
$12.95, 1-58062-670-X

Everything® **Ghost Book**
$12.95, 1-58062-533-9

Everything® **Golf Book**
$12.95, 1-55850-814-7

Everything® **Grammar and Style Book**
$12.95, 1-58062-573-8

Everything® **Guide to Las Vegas**
$12.95, 1-58062-438-3

Everything® **Guide to New England**
$12.95, 1-58062-589-4

Everything® **Guide to New York City**
$12.95, 1-58062-314-X

Everything® **Guide to Walt Disney World®,
Universal Studios®, and
Greater Orlando, 2nd Edition**
$12.95, 1-58062-404-9

Everything® **Guide to Washington D.C.**
$12.95, 1-58062-313-1

Everything® **Guitar Book**
$12.95, 1-58062-555-X

Everything® **Herbal Remedies Book**
$12.95, 1-58062-331-X

Everything® **Home-Based Business Book**
$12.95, 1-58062-364-6

Everything® **Homebuying Book**
$12.95, 1-58062-074-4

Everything® **Homeselling Book**
$12.95, 1-58062-304-2

Everything® **Horse Book**
$12.95, 1-58062-564-9

Everything® **Hot Careers Book**
$12.95, 1-58062-486-3

Everything® **Internet Book**
$12.95, 1-58062-073-6

Everything® **Investing Book**
$12.95, 1-58062-149-X

Everything® **Jewish Wedding Book**
$12.95, 1-55850-801-5

Everything® **Job Interview Book**
$12.95, 1-58062-493-6

Everything® **Lawn Care Book**
$12.95, 1-58062-487-1

Everything® **Leadership Book**
$12.95, 1-58062-513-4

Everything® **Learning French Book**
$12.95, 1-58062-649-1

Everything® **Learning Spanish Book**
$12.95, 1-58062-575-4

Everything® **Low-Fat High-Flavor Cookbook**
$12.95, 1-55850-802-3

Everything® **Magic Book**
$12.95, 1-58062-418-9

Everything® **Managing People Book**
$12.95, 1-58062-577-0

Everything® **Microsoft® Word 2000 Book**
$12.95, 1-58062-306-9

Everything® **Money Book**
$12.95, 1-58062-145-7

Everything® **Mother Goose Book**
$12.95, 1-58062-490-1

Everything® **Motorcycle Book**
$12.95, 1-58062-554-1

Everything® **Mutual Funds Book**
$12.95, 1-58062-419-7

Everything® **One-Pot Cookbook**
$12.95, 1-58062-186-4

Everything® **Online Business Book**
$12.95, 1-58062-320-4

Everything® **Online Genealogy Book**
$12.95, 1-58062-402-2

Everything® **Online Investing Book**
$12.95, 1-58062-338-7

Everything® **Online Job Search Book**
$12.95, 1-58062-365-4

Everything® **Organize Your Home Book**
$12.95, 1-58062-617-3

Everything® **Pasta Book**
$12.95, 1-55850-719-1

Everything® **Philosophy Book**
$12.95, 1-58062-644-0

Everything® **Playing Piano and Keyboards Book**
$12.95, 1-58062-651-3

Everything® **Pregnancy Book**
$12.95, 1-58062-146-5

Everything® **Pregnancy Organizer**
$15.00, 1-58062-336-0

Everything® **Project Management Book**
$12.95, 1-58062-583-5

Everything® **Puppy Book**
$12.95, 1-58062-576-2

Everything® **Quick Meals Cookbook**
$12.95, 1-58062-488-X

Everything® **Resume Book**
$12.95, 1-58062-311-5

Everything® **Romance Book**
$12.95, 1-58062-566-5

Everything® **Running Book**
$12.95, 1-58062-618-1

Everything® **Sailing Book, 2nd Edition**
$12.95, 1-58062-671-8

Everything® **Saints Book**
$12.95, 1-58062-534-7

Everything® **Selling Book**
$12.95, 1-58062-319-0

Everything® **Shakespeare Book**
$12.95, 1-58062-591-6

Everything® **Spells and Charms Book**
$12.95, 1-58062-532-0

Everything® **Start Your Own Business Book**
$12.95, 1-58062-650-5

Everything® **Stress Management Book**
$12.95, 1-58062-578-9

Everything® **Study Book**
$12.95, 1-55850-615-2

Everything® **Tai Chi and QiGong Book**
$12.95, 1-58062-646-7

Everything® **Tall Tales, Legends, and Outrageous Lies Book**
$12.95, 1-58062-514-2

Everything® **Tarot Book**
$12.95, 1-58062-191-0

Everything® **Time Management Book**
$12.95, 1-58062-492-8

Everything® **Toasts Book**
$12.95, 1-58062-189-9

Everything® **Toddler Book**
$12.95, 1-58062-592-4

Everything® **Total Fitness Book**
$12.95, 1-58062-318-2

Everything® **Trivia Book**
$12.95, 1-58062-143-0

Everything® **Tropical Fish Book**
$12.95, 1-58062-343-3

Everything® **Vegetarian Cookbook**
$12.95, 1-58062-640-8

Everything® **Vitamins, Minerals, and Nutritional Supplements Book**
$12.95, 1-58062-496-0

Everything® **Wedding Book, 2nd Edition**
$12.95, 1-58062-190-2

Everything® **Wedding Checklist**
$7.95, 1-58062-456-1

Everything® **Wedding Etiquette Book**
$7.95, 1-58062-454-5

Everything® **Wedding Organizer**
$15.00, 1-55850-828-7

Everything® **Wedding Shower Book**
$7.95, 1-58062-188-0

Everything® **Wedding Vows Book**
$7.95, 1-58062-455-3

Everything® **Weight Training Book**
$12.95, 1-58062-593-2

Everything® **Wine Book**
$12.95, 1-55850-808-2

Everything® **World War II Book**
$12.95, 1-58062-572-X

Everything® **World's Religions Book**
$12.95, 1-58062-648-3

Everything® **Yoga Book**
$12.95, 1-58062-594-0

Visit us at everything.com

Everything® is a registered trademark of Adams Media Corporation.

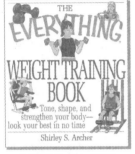